RIDE FASTER WITH LESS TIME IN THE SADDLE

RIDE FASTER WITH LESS TIME IN THE SADDLE

LEARN HOW TO IMPROVE YOUR PERSONAL RECORDS (PR'S) WITHOUT COUNTLESS HOURS OF TRAINING

LORRI ZENONI, DrPh

Copyright © 2020 Lorri C. Zenoni, DrPh
All rights reserved.
ISBN- 9798551618003

About the Author

I know what it is like to want to get faster on the bike, without additional training time. I first started riding a road bike in 2010 after my husband went on his first road bike trip and came back hooked.

I knew I wanted to get a road bike so we could ride together. I did not have lots of time to devote to riding my bike but wanted to know how I could improve my skills on the bike, while holding down a full-time job and have quality time with my husband, family and friends.

I originally created a version of this plan for myself to follow.

His 7-day bike ride would take us on a whirlwind of a bike life adventure. We would travel to Europe, ride on the same course as the Tour de France (during the TdF) and meet professional cyclists.

We started our own cycling race team for injured service members and even started a non-profit to host cycling and nutrition camps for other injured service members and veterans across the United States.

We raced both local and national events, even racing 24-hour events. I've held a World Record and we created the largest military veteran race team in the State. All from one 7-day bike ride.

The amazing thing is that I did ALL of this while holding down a full-time job. I was not a full-time cyclist yet was able to ride and compete like one. The plan that you see in this book is years of revisions to keep my own fitness up, while enjoying my life off the bike.

I have decided to share it with you, so you can make the most gains, with the time you have to spend on the bike. While we are all different and respond to gains individually, the information in here can be applied to most cyclists.

Dr. Lorri Zenoni, DrPh

Acknowledgements

This book is dedicated to my husband, Dean. (The sexy one on the cover). It is

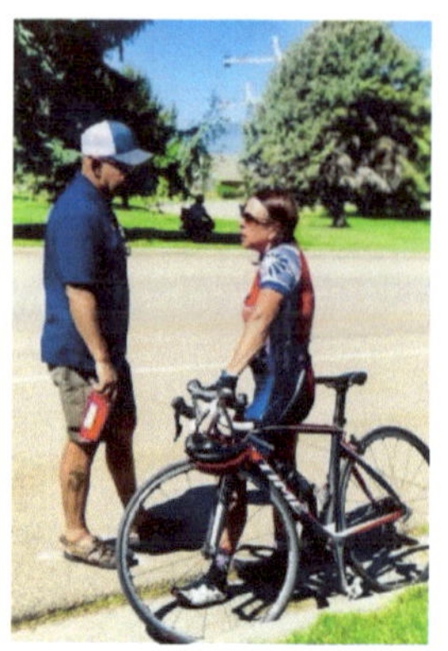 because of his love and support that I was able to ride my bike and compete like a champion, while still maintaining a household and a career. He is my mechanic, my bike builder, my wheel builder (he even made me carbon wheels with our last name on it). He is my coach, my cheerleader, my riding partner, my sounding board and my reality check.
He is the LOVE of my life and none of this would have been possible without his unwavering support and love. I can't wait to see where our adventures take us next. All my love!

I also want to give some other shout outs to those who have made this book possible. Photo Credits go out to Frazer Hazlett for the amazing cover photo taken during the Hoodoo 500 race that we crewed ourselves for 500 miles in 3 days. We were either riding or driving, and while Frazer was Crew Chief Extraordinaire for our cycle mates, he was able to capture this glorious shot.

Photo Credit to Candice Snow for the continual support during the Project Hero challenges. She was always in the right spot at the right time, with a smile. Photo Credit to Robyn Noel for her wicked strong attitude, amazing dedication to our team and the tenacity to never quit.

To our local race team that inspired me to show up every week and give it my all. To my fellow racers and competitors who taught me the ins and outs of racing competitively.

To the club and recreational cyclists for your dedication to the sport that has allowed me to learn from you and continue to make this a better sport for all. To the cycling groups that we have traveled with to some amazing adventures. Thank you for the memories that will last a lifetime.

My bicycle has allowed me to see the world. I have met some of the most amazing people while on my bike. I am in awe of what a 7-Day Bicycle event has done for our lives and those we have met. Here's to many more bicycling adventures.

Contents

Introduction

Congratulations and thank you for buying this book. If you are a cyclist that has a career and/or a family yet wants to improve your performance on your bike without countless hours spent on the bike, then this book is for you.

The information in this book is provided for educational and/or informational purposes only. It is not intended to be a substitute for professional medical advice, diagnosis or treatment. Always seek the advice of your qualified healthcare provider with any questions you may have regarding a medical condition. Never disregard professional medical advice or delay seeking medical care because of something you have read in this book.

Let's step back and look at your own journey on your bike. You started out with your first bike and you have made great progress since day one. You found a local cycling club/group to start riding with and others who were at your same level of riding. You have gotten the hang of the bike and have ridden your way up to the middle of the pack and even further.

You even found a few cycling friends that you look forward to riding with. You schedule rides with these new friends outside the club and you are having fun. You love to feel the wind on your face and at your back. You only wish you had found this sport earlier in life.

You start improving your PR's on your favorite rides. You didn't think you would care about PR's, but you have become a little obsessed. Your competitive nature is coming out. You come home and instantly download your ride to your favorite exercise tracking network or cycling head unit. It keeps track of how well you did as well as compares you to others in your same age and gender category. You start to collect badges the more you ride, and you are motivated by your progress.

You have started to increase the amount of time you spend on your bike. You come home from work and ride before it gets dark. You have figured out how to ride this weekend with the club ride around your family time. You even take your bike to work to fit in a short ride at lunch.

You are starting to wonder if you can keep improving your performance, but not have to keep increasing your bike time?

You have gone from riding 1-3 hours a week to riding upwards of 5-7 hours a week. Riding your bike is your stress release and you absolutely love it. But you also realize that your family time or work is suffering. The biking world is an exciting place to get fit and have fun, but you wonder if you can have the best of both worlds?

After 10 years on the bike, I am excited to share these lifestyle tips with you that I used to create more fun and speed on the bike, without sacrificing my job and life off the bike. It also created more experiences and adventures. Just a caveat. This book does not contain training plans. This book is dedicated to improving your performance on your bike by improving your health.

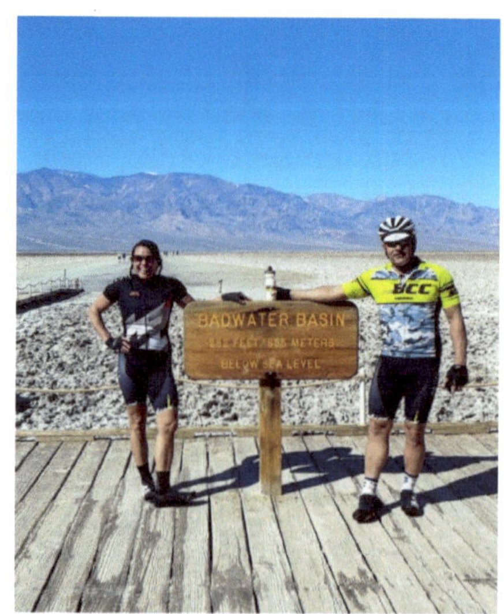

Death Valley National Park-BadWater Basin

Can You Really Get Faster Without More Training Time in the Saddle?

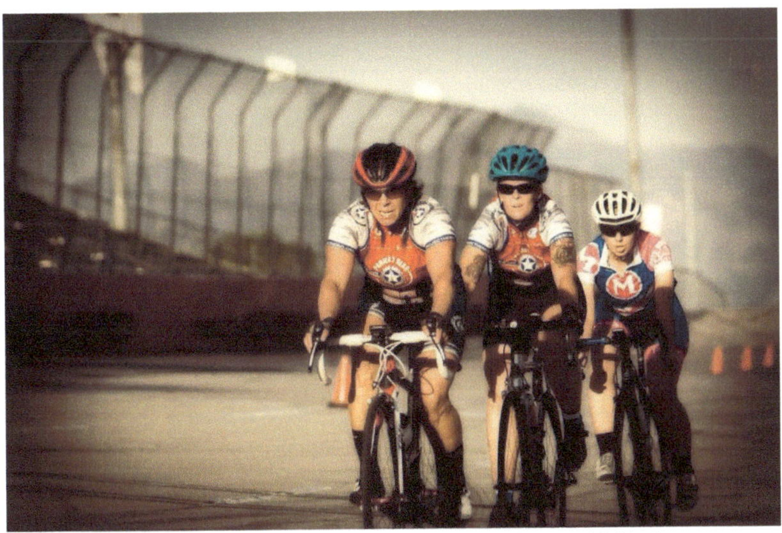

Criterium Racing in Utah at RMR Oval Track

What if you could improve your PR's without adding extra riding hours to your week?

As you talk with club riders and ask the stronger riders how many hours, they ride a week, they share that they ride 4-5 days a week, 10-12 hours a week with the club. They may even add another training ride in, depending on the week.

You want to be as strong and fast as them to keep up, but you know you can't dedicate that many days or hours a week to riding. You have a family. You have a job. You are not a full-time cyclist. You have responsibilities that won't allow you to ride that much, even though you may want to ride that much. It is just not possible for you.

You start to think the only way to improve your PR's is to increase your riding days and the length of your rides. You start to accept that you will have to remain at the level you are at, because you just can't give up that much time to ride a bike.

You can't possibly justify "improving your PR's" in exchange for partner or family time.

You want to live a balanced life with both peak performance and a healthy life off the bike. You start to wonder if this is even possible?

What if I told you there was a way? What if you could have the best of both worlds? What if you could improve your PR's without adding extra riding hours to your week? What if living a balanced life is possible? If this sounds like you, then you are in the right place. This book was written with you in mind.

I have spent the last 10 years improving upon this plan you see in this book. I am a lifelong learner and have educated myself through school, certificates and continual learning. I have a degree in nutrition, certificates in sports nutrition and even a doctorate in Preventive Care and Lifestyle Medicine. I don't tell you this to brag, but to let you know that this book is not based on "bro science" or an influencer's anecdotal advice but is based on nutrition and lifestyle science and proven results.

Let's Make a Deal

These strategies are easy to implement, yet easy not to implement.

I am going to outline 3 proven strategies for you to improve your performance on the bike without additional training time in the saddle. These strategies are easy to implement, yet easy not to implement. Some of you may think they seem too easy to do and you won't do them. Or you are already doing most of them, so you don't take this seriously. Others may also look at them as too much to do. Wherever you fall on this spectrum, commit to make daily changes.

Make yourself a promise. You invested in this book, which means you made a commitment to invest in yourself. Make a promise to yourself that you will follow these simple strategies for a minimum of 30 days. Make a promise to yourself that no matter how easy it may be to do these things, that you will still do them. Truly commit to yourself and follow this plan.

There is something in here for everyone to work on. If you are already doing many of these tips, then focus on the ones you are not doing.

Or focus on mastering the ones you are already performing. Some of you may have more tasks than others to work on but focus first on the strategies that you are performing and do them a little bit better. Then, focus on the strategies that you are not doing and keep improving day by day. There is always room to improve on these strategies, no matter which stage you are in.

In general, I have found that most Cat 1 & 2 riders have their plan dialed in. It is the Cat 3, 4 & 5's, along with club riders that are really looking for a plan. If this is you, there is definitely something in this book for you.

For every person that buys this book, I will also do a check-in with you in 30 days. When I message you on the private Facebook page, I want to hear how this program has helped you and how many seconds and minutes you have shaved off your favorite ride. I want to hear about your favorite ride and your pre and post time on this ride. I want to hear how this book has helped you and what you have discovered about yourself and your bike journey.

Make a commitment that when I reach out to you, you have a success story to share with me. I don't want you to be the one that ignores me because you did not implement these simple strategies. Deal? Say it out loud for those in the back, **DEAL!**

"A little progress each day, adds up to big results. "

unknown

Getting Started

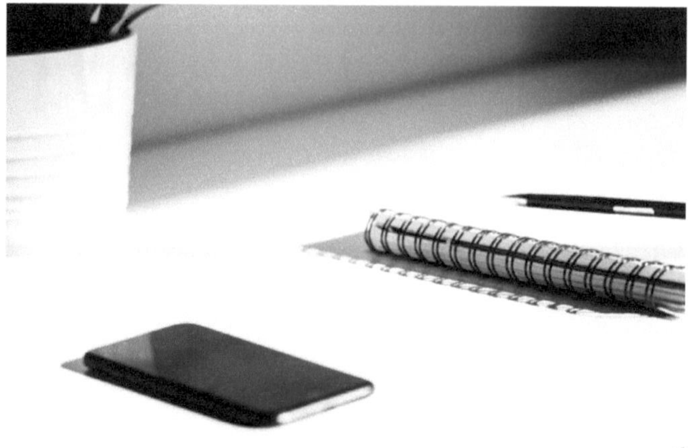

First, before we get to the strategies, let's make sure you have a tracking system to use to measure your PR's. We need a way to see if your PR's are improving. If you use an exercise tracking system or an app on your phone, that is great to keep your data. But I would still like you to use a spreadsheet to transfer the data from your tracking system to the spreadsheet.

I know this is old school. But it keeps your times top of mind. It allows you to easily access your times and even show them to a friend or family member, if you want to brag on yourself. (And trust me, as those times improve, you will want to sing it out loud.)

As you may know, there are many segments that can be tracked on your exercise tracking system. To start, pick a few that you would be proud of if they improved. Look through your tracking system and see where you already have a PR.

Or find a segment that is more challenging for you and you want to learn to ride that segment faster and stronger. Once you find those segments, put them in a notebook or on a spreadsheet.

If you use a notebook or a spreadsheet, use these minimum criteria to track.

Name of Segment

Your Time

Date of Record

List the name of the 2-3 segments that you want to track first. Your tracking device may have them already named or maybe you have a special name for that segment. You may add more segments than that eventually but pick 2-3 to start. Pick segments that you really want to improve upon, then add the date that you made that record. Lastly, post your time of your record.

You are welcome to add more items to track, such as external conditions (wind, rain, tailwind, headwind, extreme heat, rode with a group, etc.), internal conditions (how did you feel that day, had a great night's sleep, didn't eat before my ride, etc.), but the three items listed above are the basics needed.

I would then suggest that you attempt to ride those segments at least once a week. To see how your times are improving as you follow the strategies outlined in this book. Each time you ride the segments, you would record your new time and date on your tracker.

On the next page is an example of a simple spreadsheet to keep track of your records. Nothing fancy. Just a way to record your personal records. I made this spreadsheet in Excel.

Sample PR Tracker

Name of Segment	Current time	Date
Name of Segment	Current time	Date
Name of Segment	Current time	Date
Name of Segment	Current time	Date

This is a simple Excel document that you can re-create to track your segments that you will work on improving. You could also create this as a table in Microsoft Word or use a notebook. You may add other columns if you want to keep track of other data, but this will be the minimum information to track.

Now on to the Strategies. The reason you bought this book.

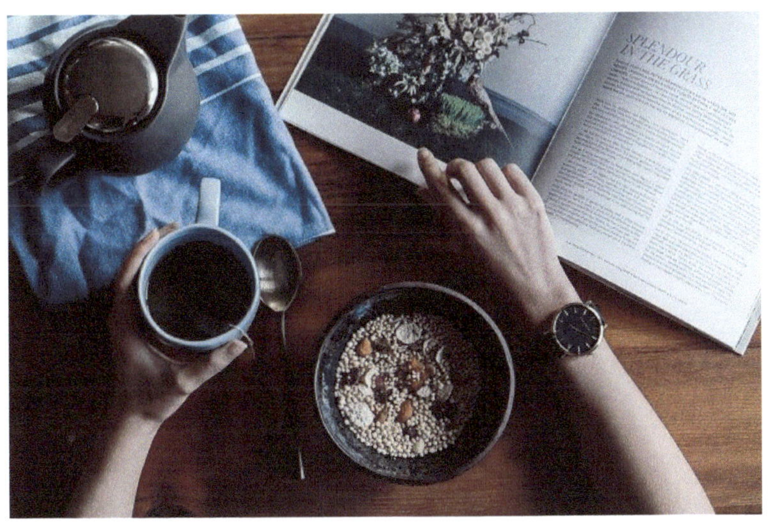

STRATEGY #1

Eat Healthier OFF the Bike

What does this mean? It means that everything you eat, and drink is focused on the healthier end of the spectrum. It means we eat more foods that provide us with vitamins and minerals and nutrients and less foods that just provide us with empty calories.

Empty calories mean there are no real benefits (vitamins, minerals) to these foods. We just eat or drink empty calories but may not nourish our body from these calories. A good example of empty calories is soda.) Now, those of you that love soda, please don't put up a roadblock yet. There can be a time and place for it.)

While healthy means something different to each one of us, as cyclists we may know which foods work better in our body and which ones wreak havoc on our systems.

Eating healthier means you treat your body with respect when it comes to food. You start thinking about what food can do for your body, not just how it tastes.

Don't misunderstand me here, as healthy food should also taste good. Eating healthy is not tasteless, you may just need to retrain your taste buds.

For the next 30 days, I am suggesting you repeat the following affirmation, "Food is my Strength". Wake up every morning for the next 30 days and tell yourself "Food is my Strength" before you get out of bed.

Everything you put into your body is to help your body get stronger on the bike. It is to help you lead a healthier life as well as improve your personal records. We have to eat food anyway and knowing you can make easy gains for not much effort is a relief to most cyclists.

Over the next 30 days, let's focus on a new way of thinking about food.

***Think the food you eat is to strengthen your body.**

***Think the food you eat is fuel for your body.**

***Think the food you eat is to nourish your body from head to toe.**

When we think of food as our support and friend on the bike, we can look at the way we eat differently. This includes both on and off the bike. This first strategy will focus OFF the bike. We will focus on how we eat on any given day. I know there are days when you are not cooking, or you are at a friend's home, and these principles can still apply.

I also know you are probably not the only person that you are making food for in your home. Or maybe you don't do the cooking. That is okay! Each of these principles can also be applied to your family and still work.

Your family may not be as willing to try them as you are but ask them to support you over the next 30 days. Let them know you are on a mission to improve your times on your bike, without taking away additional time from them. Ask them if they can support you in this mission.

Go over all these strategies and tasks with them, so they know exactly how they will support you. Ask them if they will be a member of your support team. Ask them if they will be a part of your SAG (support and gear) team.

They have most likely already volunteered to be on your SAG team for other events and trainings but may not have been officially asked or knew their role. For the most part, your partner and family members like to help.

Let them know this is a time when you need their support. Let them know you are on a new plan for the next 30 days. Our team likes to know how long we are asking them to support us for a given event.

Once your team is in place, you're READY to take on your tasks.

Coming Together is a beginning,
Staying Together is progress,
Working Together is success.

Henry Ford

Here are your Tasks to Start Eating Healthier OFF the bike:

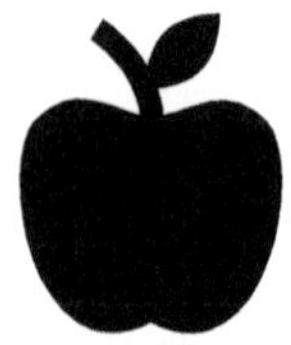

Your Strategy #1 tasks to eat healthier OFF your bike.

- Eat more fruits and vegetables
- Aim for eating protein at each meal, every day
- Try one new vegetable each week
- Reduce fast food visits to no more than once a week
- Reduce soda and sweetened drinks
- Increase or maintain water intake to half of your body weight in ounces
- Eat regularly throughout the day
- Eat Slowly

Now, let's break them down, one by one. Let's discuss how to accomplish these tasks.

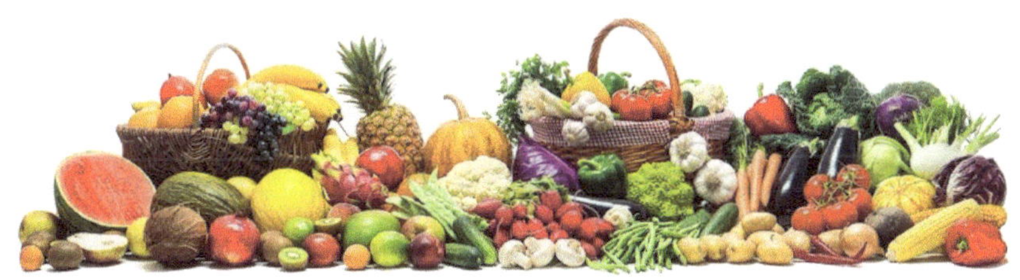

Task #1-Eat more fruits and vegetables daily

This task simply involves eating more fruits and vegetables on a daily basis. Fruits and vegetables provide more fiber, vitamins, minerals and micronutrients that your body may be lacking.

They also provide more water to your body. Fruits and vegetables have other health benefits as well by keeping your appetite in check. They are quick and easy to eat and are available almost everywhere you shop.

Aim for a fruit or vegetable at every meal and even as snacks. For example, if you have an egg sandwich for breakfast, add a little spinach in the eggs while cooking. Or in your protein shake, mix in some blueberries or a banana. Fruit is actually easy to have as a snack both on and off the bike. It is easy to stuff a banana in your jersey pocket and have it at your halfway point.

Try to eat fruits and vegetables that are in season as they will taste better and will be more economical. Look for sales at the grocery store and take advantage of stocking up on items you and your family will eat. If something is on sale, can you buy now and freeze for later?

You may even look into a fruit and vegetable cooperative that will allow you to order a basket of seasonal fruits and vegetables at a discounted community price. I love to buy from food co-ops, so do a search in your area and see if you have one in your neighborhood.

Have you heard the term, "Eat the Rainbow"? There is a rainbow of colors in the produce aisle and these colors provide us with micronutrients (vitamins and minerals) and phytonutrients (natural chemicals in plants, that may act as antioxidants or anti-inflammatories). In this first task, we want to get more color on our plates and focus on eating the rainbow every day.

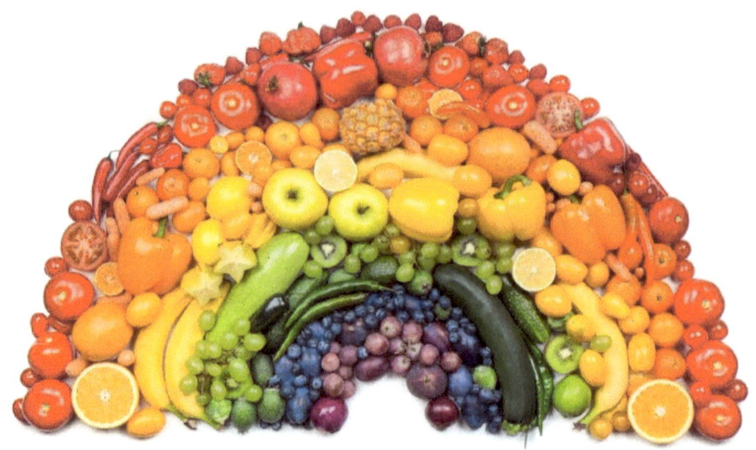

When fruit and vegetables look this good and taste fresh, you are more likely to eat them and eat more of them. You can even challenge yourself during these first 30 days to see if you can try different colors. Maybe you set a few color themes for the day.

For example, you can make it a green, orange and purple day and add those colors to your meal. For example, you would have green spinach, orange tomato and purple carrots in your salad. You can get your family or kids involved and ask them to pick a color for the day or the week.

Make it fun and make it taste good. Food is meant to be enjoyed and fresh colors with fresh tastes give flavor and fun to your meals.

While our goal is to eat fresh, when possible, you may need to eat frozen or in a can. Frozen, would be the next best option as there is usually less sugar or preservatives added. Canned would be the last choice.

If canned is your only option, choose fruits packed in their own juice and less sugar. For vegetables, you can buy the low sodium varieties or rinse the vegetables with water before eating to rid them of the extra sodium packed in the can.

How do you save fruit and vegetables from being tossed out?
Fruits and vegetables taste best when they are fresh and in season. Sometimes we buy fresh fruits and vegetables and then don't use them in time.
Here are a few tips to save them-
1. Blend them in the blender in your favorite smoothie.
2. Blend fruit together with some ice to make a frozen treat.
3. Cut up the vegetables and make a soup or stew.
4. Cut up and put in a freezer safe bag and use for later in smoothies, soups or stews or salsas. Some of my favorite fruits to freeze are bananas, berries (blueberries, strawberries, blackberries), mangos and cherries. My favorite vegetables to freeze are green beans, zucchini, squash, tomatoes, (I make salsa or sauce with them and then freeze that).

I love knowing that I am getting the nutrients that I can from these foods and not tossing them.

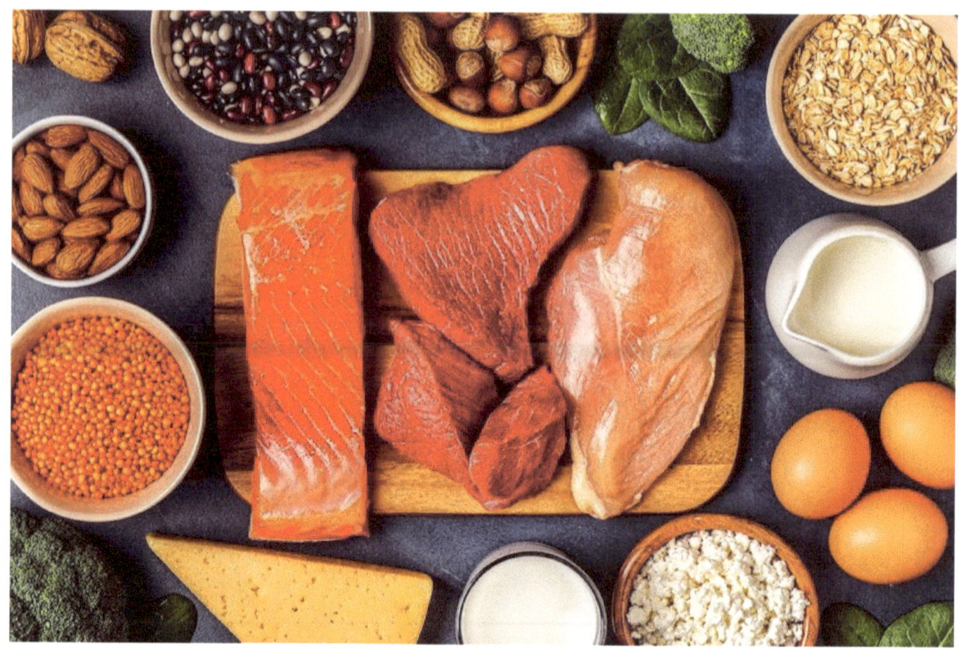

Task #2- Aim for eating protein at each meal

The importance of protein for athletes has long been recognized. Protein is one of your body's most powerful macronutrients and is made up of building blocks, called amino acids. While there are several studies and different recommendations of exact ingestion, it depends on your activity and the individual.

As this is a basic guide to improving your nutrition, we will focus on eating protein at every meal, instead of an exact number of grams. (Although we will discuss suggested number of grams in the follow-up for those of you that are ready to take it to the next step).

Protein plays a key role in the creation and maintenance of every cell in our body. As a cyclist, eating protein daily is important for building lean muscle and reducing muscle loss. This is important as we aim to improve our personal records. Protein can also assist to speed up recovery after exercise and/or injury.

We want to make sure our muscles are working to their maximum effort and protein will help us to improve our PR's without more time on the bike.

Which foods have quality protein in them? Lean meats (chicken, beef, turkey, pork), fish and seafood, eggs, protein powder, dairy products, beans, peas and legumes, lentils, oats, nuts and seeds.

Many vegetables also have protein, we just have to eat more of them to get adequate intake. Table 5 provides the protein content in common foods. When cooking meats, focus on leaner cuts or trim off the visible fat. Grilling or baking is suggested over frying.

Use your palm as a guide on how much to eat. In general, for males, aim for 2 palms per meal. For females, aim for one palm per meal. This is a general guideline and you may need more or less depending on your individual needs. This does not mean that men need twice as much food as women, or that women need half as much food as men, these are just simple appropriations. Based on your individual needs, you may need more or less than this recommendation.

If you need more individualized planning, sign up on our wait list for our course "The Fuel Playbook." This 6-week course is specific to the Endurance Athlete and provides proven strategies to help you unlock the power of nutrition to optimize your athletic performance. This course is based on real science, and will help you boost your endurance, take out the frustration of knowing exactly what to eat and when and help you have more energy on and off the road.

We only release this course twice a year. If you want to be on the wait list for this course, send an email to drlorriz@thefueltrainer.com and put "The Fuel Playbook Wait List" in the Subject Line.

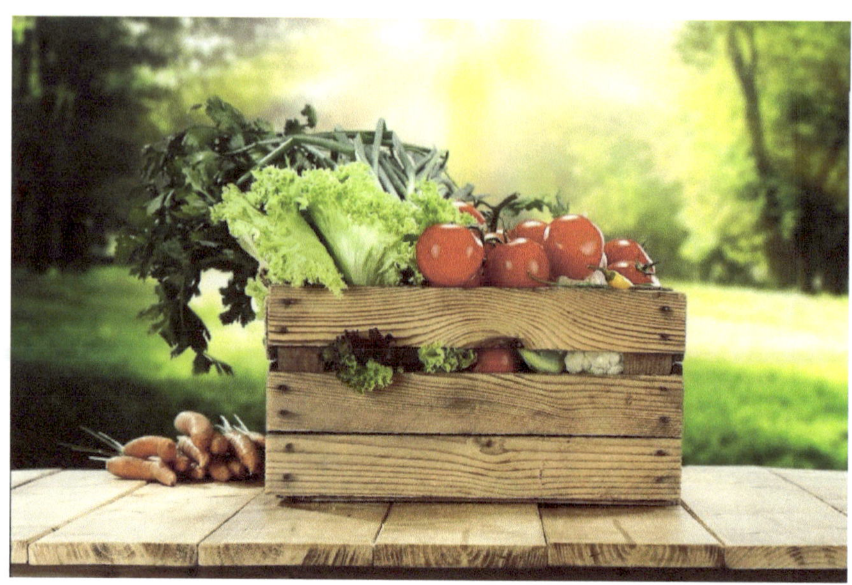

Task #3- Try a new vegetable each week

Vegetables provide us with vitamins, minerals and micronutrients. Most of society is deficient in micronutrients and don't even know it. Some statistics even state that 80% of society is deficient in micronutrients. As we look to improve our PR's, it will be important to get more micronutrients into our body so our bodies can perform at an optimal level.

What are your favorite vegetables? How often do you eat them? Make a list of the vegetables that you normally eat and ones you have wanted to try. Think about 4 new vegetables that you will try over the next 30 days.

Go to the store and look around in the produce section. Look at something that you have never eaten and then figure out a way to make it in a recipe. Do a search on the internet for possible recipes for that vegetable. It doesn't have to be exotic, just something you have not eaten before. Maybe it is cauliflower or asparagus or arugula?

Recipe Tip Idea

I love to put raw vegetables on a sheet pan and roast them in the oven. I coat them with a little olive oil and sea salt and put them in the standard oven for about 20-25 minutes at 400 degrees, depending on the type of vegetables on my pan. I love to put broccoli, cauliflower, Brussel sprouts, mushrooms, carrots, onions and sweet potatoes (cut in chunks) on my sheet pan. Here is a picture before cooking.

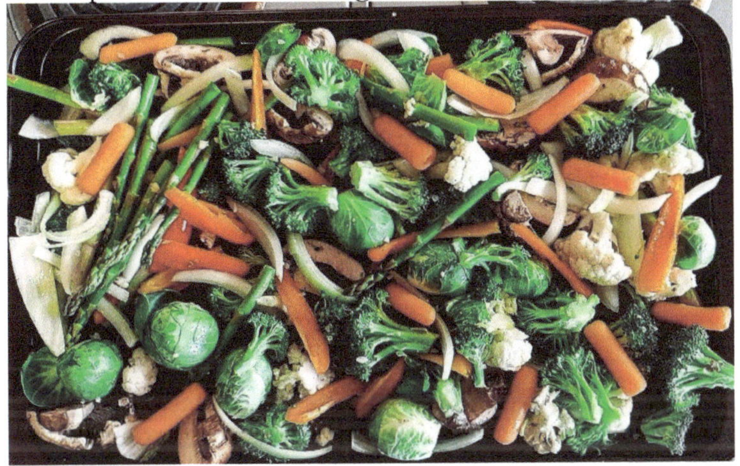

You can even find a new recipe for a vegetable that you have already eaten or cook it a different way. Spice up the way you eat vegetables with herbs and spices and not with sauces or creams. Sauces, butter and creams can add extra saturated fat and calories that are not needed. You can cook them lightly in olive oil and sea salt but try to reduce any other extra calories on your vegetables.

Pick vegetables that are in season and naturally ripe. Visit a Farmer's Market for local produce. At a Farmer's Market, you will learn that all vegetables do not look perfect, like they do at a grocery store. But they taste so much better.

Learn to enjoy the taste of vegetables and aim for at least 5 servings a day. As a reference, you can use your fist as a serving of vegetables. With this reference, aim for at least 5 fists each day, with one new vegetable a week.

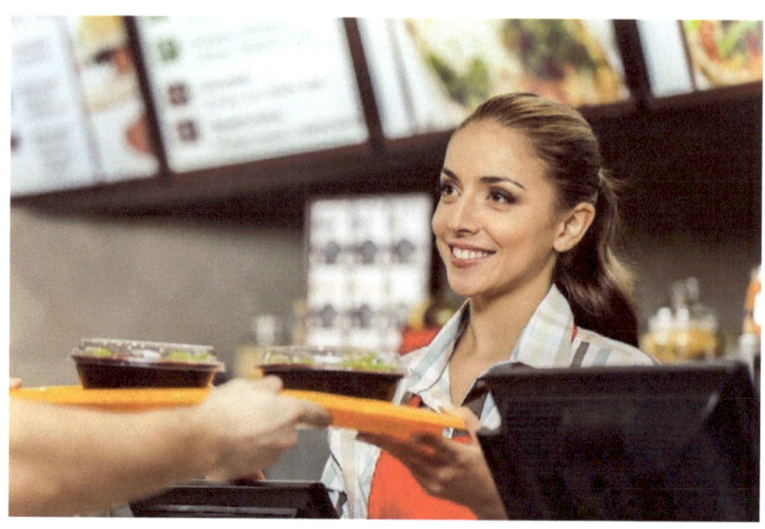

Task #4-Reduce fast food visits to no more than once per week

Most fast foods are full of saturated fat and calories. One meal can easily add up to over half your daily intake of calories and almost your whole day's allotment of fat. I know fast food is quick and easy, especially if you are running late somewhere or did not plan a meal. But, for the next 30 days, let's plan to reduce your fast food visits to no more than once per week.

If you need help to plan your meal so you don't run to your favorite fast food window, start with time-blocking a time in the evening to make your lunch for the next day. Put it in a lunch box or small cooler to take with you during the workday. You will save money as well as calories. Plus, you will be training your body to be stronger on the bike, with less empty calories.

If you have a family that likes to visit fast food, you can also apply this principle to them. As your support team members, remind them of the mission you are all on together.

When you visit your favorite fast food establishment, keeping these tips in mind may help.

1. **Keep portion sizes small.** Order the kids size portion or split a meal with a partner. In general, when we eat out, portion sizes are much larger than we need. We tend to think we get more value for our food, if the portion size is larger. Larger portion sizes may not be best for our health. A larger portion does not mean we need to eat everything on our plate. Share a meal or take some home, if you can.
2. **Choose a healthier side dish.** Choose the side salad, a plain baked potato or apple slices.
3. **Go for the greens.** Many fast foods now have specialty salads. Just watch the extra dressing and cheese that add saturated fat and calories. If you order the dressing on the side, you can dip your fork in the dressing when you take a bite. You will still get the flavor and taste of the dressing, without soaking your salad in it.
4. **Watch out for high-calorie salads**-a taco salad in a crispy shell can add an extra 1000 calories to your day.
5. **Skip high fat salad extras**- some of these gourmet salads are loaded with cheese, croutons, toppings (sour cream) and dressings. Ask for these items to be removed or order on the side.
6. **Opt for grilled items**-a grilled choice will have less calories and less fat.
7. **Watch your drink**-a large soda (32 ounces) has about 300 empty calories. A large shake has about 800 calories and all of a day's allotment from saturated fat. Choose water, with lemon if you need flavoring, when you can. If you want carbonation, go for sparkling water or mineral water. Studies show that those who drink "diet drinks" tend to eat more. My number one go to drink I recommend is water.

Some have said that these tips "take the fun out of eating at fast food". My response is to weigh the benefits of this food on your goal. Does eating here move you closer or further away from your goals? Once you have the answer to this question for your own goals, then you have more motivation when eating quick, fast food.

If "Food is your Strength", ask yourself if this fast food gives you strength? The other way to look at this is through the perspective of moderation and healthy balance. If you follow these tips for 2 of your 4 trips this month, then on the other visits, you can eat what you want at your favorite establishment. That's what I call a Win-Win.

When you do visit a fast food establishment, make it intentional. Plan in advance what you are going to eat there.

If you get stuck out and you need to grab a quick bite to eat, here are some options that may be healthier than others. This list is not exhaustive, just a few options.

- An omelet with veggies of your choice and no cheese (or half cheese)
- A bowl of oatmeal with fruit and nuts as toppings
- Scrambled eggs with vegetables and whole grain toast
- A grilled chicken sandwich, no mayo. A la carte.
- A burger wrapped in lettuce or a whole wheat bun. Skip the fries.
- A grilled chicken or steak burrito with no cheese or sour cream.
- A rice bowl with grilled meat and stir-fry veggies. Ask for half the sauce.
- Flame-grilled chicken with beans and rice.
- A tomato-based soup with half a sandwich.
- A roast turkey salad with an oil and vinegar dressing on the side.
- A rotisserie chicken from the grocery store with a pre-made green salad. (this would have leftovers and may need a cooler to take home with you)

- A grilled chicken wrap with no mayo. Load up on the spinach and veggies.
- A grilled meat burrito bowl with salsa and no tortilla.
- A specialty apple and chicken salad, with dressing on the side.
- Lettuce wraps with grilled chicken or grilled steak.

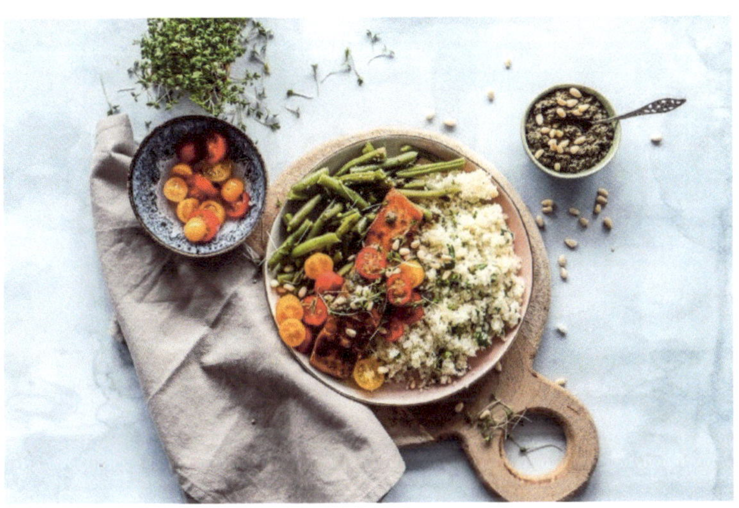

A salmon bowl with quinoa

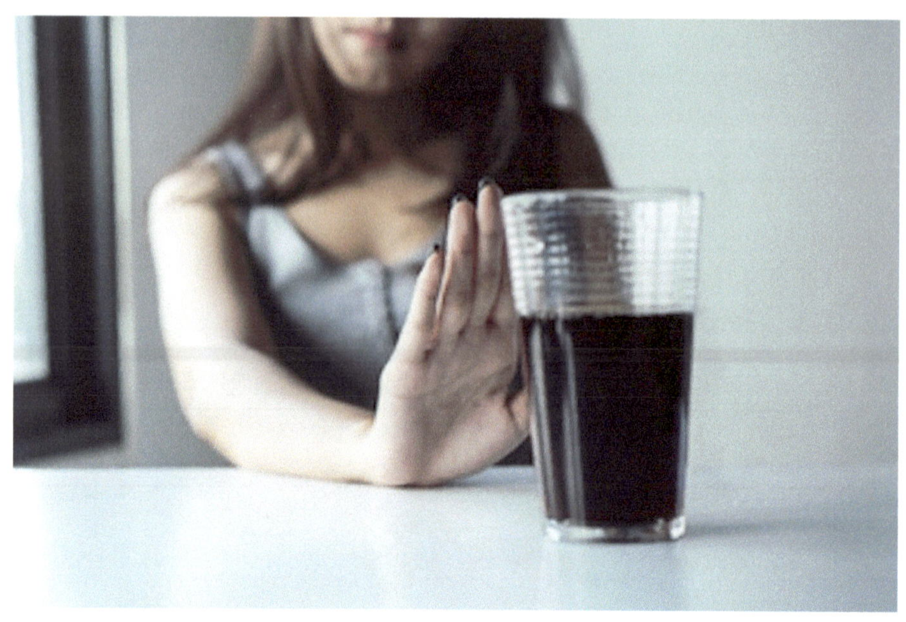

Task #5-Reduce soda and sweetened drinks

Soda is full of sugar. As a matter of fact, it is often called "liquid sugar". It is a drink full of empty calories. Soda and sugary drinks are the single largest source of calories and added sugar in the U.S. diet. Did you know that a 12 ounce can of soda can have over 10 spoons of sugar in it? Would you take a glass of water and put 10 spoons of sugar in it and drink it? Most of us would not.

These calories do not provide you with nutrients and yet can provide you with a sugar overload. Although your muscles love carbohydrates, this is not the type of carbohydrate that will fuel your muscles to improve your PR's. When you drink sugary calories, you do not feel as full as you would if you had eaten those calories. Again, another source of wasted calories.

When consuming more processed sugar (found in sodas and sweetened drinks), you may experience a host of ailments from digestive issues, mood issues, skin issues and weight gain.

To improve our overall health and to give our body the best fuel, reduce or eliminate soda and sugary drinks during these first 30 days. If you want some natural flavor, add fresh squeezed orange, lemon or lime to your water. Or you can try a fruit infusion with frozen berries or your favorite fruit as added flavor. Some like to put in cucumber or mint in their water.

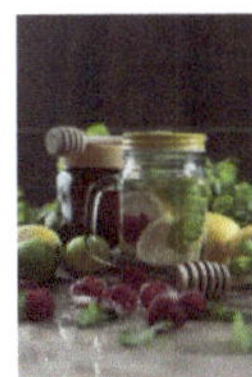

There are plenty of ways to experiment.

*Add fresh fruit and vegetables. Infusions are not the place for bruised or overly ripe pieces.

*Select your infusion mix with your favorite flavors. (Cucumber/mint, lemon/mint, triple berry delight, strawberry/basil/lemon, pineapple/coconut/lime, mango/raspberry/ginger) or try your own.

* Slice fruit and veggies thin for better flavor release.

*Infused water can be made ahead of time- 2-12 hours before drinking.

*Eating the fruit-you can eat the fruit in the water but know it may have lost its flavor in the water.

<u>Instructions</u>

In a large pitcher, place the desired combination of fruit or herbs. Add ice and fill container with water. Add additional fruit or herbs to garnish, if desired. Let sit for at least 2 hours.

Drink and Enjoy!

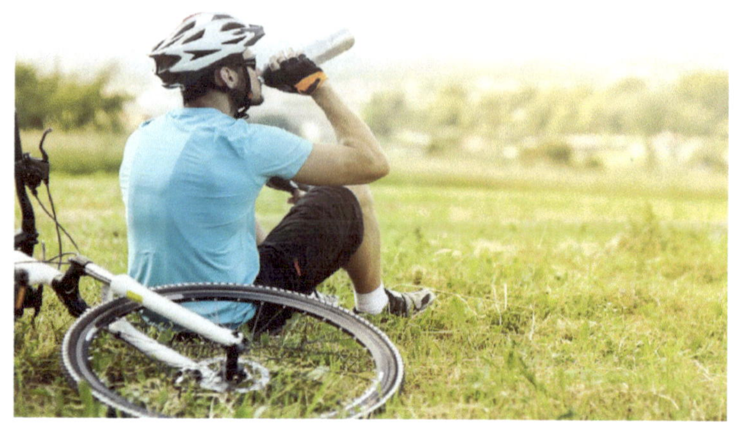

Task #6-Increase or maintain water intake to half of your body weight in ounces

The Institute of Medicine (IOM) recommends 13 cups (10.5 from beverages) for men and 9 cups (about 7 from beverages) for women. I like to recommend half of your body weight, including the water you will drink on the bike. This depends on the individual cyclist. It may be slightly different, depending on the athlete, but is a good general recommendation.

For example, if you weigh 150 pounds, aim for 75 ounces of water minimum a day. There are 8 ounces of water in one cup. If you are aiming for 75 ounces, you would drink approximately 9 cups of water. (We will talk about hydration on the bike later).

Your water intake also varies on the conditions you are in. Is it hot or humid? If it is, you may need a little more. If you are a heavy sweater, you may need more. On average, an adult loses 2-3 liters a day in sweat, urine and bowel movements. One liter is equivalent to 33.8 ounces. I usually just round this up to 34 ounces.

At a minimum, you want to replace 68-101 ounces of water.
Instead of worrying about the different #'s and to try and simplify the
process, I recommend half of your body weight for cyclists.

Water is nature's first energy drink.

When we are dehydrated, we may feel tired, dizzy, or urinate and sweat less.
For many, when they are tired, they reach for a caffeinated drink. There may
be a time and place for caffeine, but when you are tired, let's think about the
last time you drank water. Grab that container and drink up and see if you
can improve some of these symptoms.

Think about these stats when it comes to dehydration:

*If you lose 2% of your body's fluid, your overall performance will
considerably drop.

*If you lose 5% of your body's fluid, you can find yourself facing heat
exhaustion, which is not good. Now, you are barely moving.

*If you lose 10% of your body's fluid, you are at risk for heat stroke and
even death through dehydration. In other words, game over.

At 2% loss, most people don't feel it, yet are already impacting their performance.

Water provides us with cushion and lubrication for our joints. It helps us to
regulate temperature and nourishes our brain and spinal cord. Our bodies
are made up of 55-60% water and almost all of our organs are made up of at
least 1/3 -3/4 water.

There are many foods that contain water as well. Here are a few with the highest water content.

Food Name	Water Content
Lettuce	96%
Cucumber	95%
Celery	95%
Bok Choy	95%
Tomato	94%
Watermelon	92%
Cauliflower	92%
Strawberries	91%
Cantaloupe	90%
Peaches	89%
Oranges	88%

A dehydrated brain has to work harder and if you are dehydrated, you are not setting PR's. So, eat more water in your food and **drink up every day.**

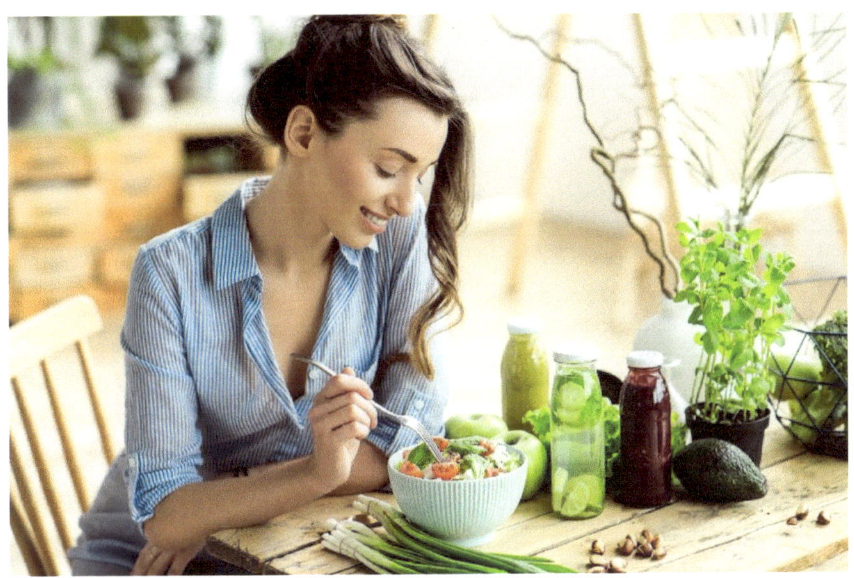

Task #7-Eat Regularly Throughout the Day

Start your day with breakfast. Breakfast is an important meal of the day. I don't call it the most important meal, as I think all meals are important. But it breaks the fast from your sleep. If you are going to ride in the morning, breakfast will be important. Think about foods that fuel your body and give you strength.

If you go too long without eating, (for most people this is 3-4 hours), your body may become fatigued or light-headed. If you are not fueled properly, you will not have enough glycogen in your muscles and will not have the strength to ride hard and fast.

What does it mean to eat regularly? While this may vary from person to person, aim for at least 3 meals a day and 1-2 snacks, depending on your lifestyle, riding schedule and caloric needs. If you are not riding that day, then you will most likely not need as much food as on the days you are riding.

Predicting energy expenditure (how many calories you burn) can be estimated with formulas. We will calculate your individual Resting Metabolic Rate (RMR), or how many calories your body burns while at rest in The Fuel Playbook course.

Some people like to eat smaller meals throughout the day. For instance, they may eat six smaller meals, instead of three larger meals. There is no one right way. How many meals you eat depends on your lifestyle, on and off the bike, and your caloric intake goal.

No matter what works for you, try to eat between 400-600 calories per meal. Any less than 400, is most likely a snack and you may be hungry in an hour or two. More than 600 calories and you may start to feel sluggish as your body is having to work harder to process and digest that meal. If you have a higher caloric daily goal, you may see the need to eat more often to stay in the 400-600 calorie meal range.

I like to use an analogy here of putting gas in your car. Most people will not get in their car and expect it to drive without gas, yet people get in their bodies all day long without "fuel" and expect that body to perform at its best. Commit to the next 30 days to fuel your body with regular, healthy meals throughout the day. If your goal is to truly improve your PR's, you will need to fuel your body regularly for this task.

Every time you eat is an opportunity to nourish your body.

Unknown

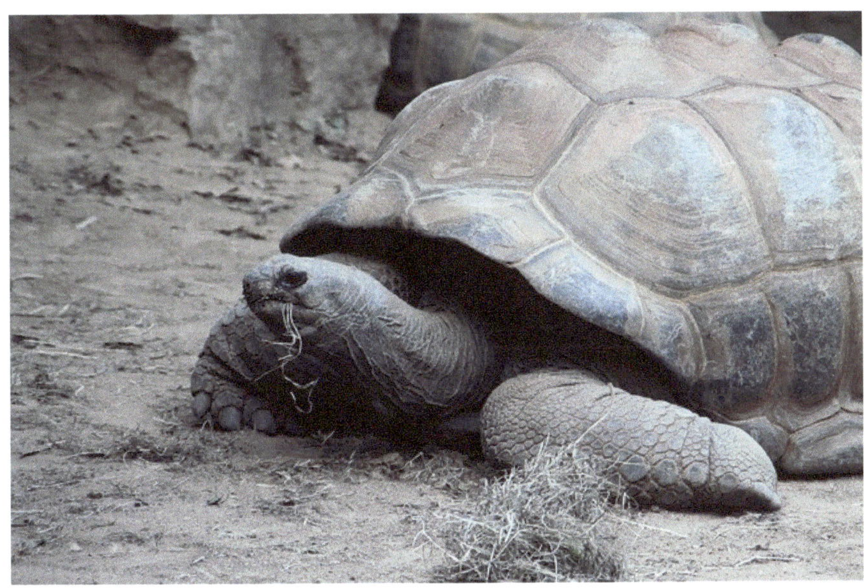

Task #8-Eat Slowly

Did you know there are studies of people eating slowly and actually taking in less calories to get full? It takes some time for our brain to get the signal from your stomach that it is full. Yet, most of us have gone back for seconds, before our brain even gets the signal. Then, we are over-stuffed and wonder how we ate so much.

This simple trick of eating slowly can help to not over-eat and eliminate that stuffed feeling.

Here is an exercise to try at your meals. Count how many chews per bite of food you can perform. Put a bite of food in your mouth and then start counting. If it is something more substantial as meat, you could potentially get up to 40 chews. If it is a soft vegetable, you may be lucky to get 10. Make it a game. You will notice when you chew your food more that you taste the flavors of the food more. It is a practice in patience also as it can be annoying for some to count their chews. But, if you do, you tend to eat less over the course of the day.

Try it out and see. Make a game at the dinner table with your kids or partner.

There they are. The 8 tasks that you will practice over the next 30 days. The 8 tasks in Strategy #1 that will move you closer to improving your PR's on your bike, without adding extra training hours on your bike.

As I stated in the beginning, these may seem simple for some and harder for others. If this list seems too overwhelming, then step back and look at which tasks you are already successful at. Or, which tasks seem easier for you to accomplish. Start with those and once those are mastered, move on to the next task. If you need to break them into baby steps, then do it.

I suggest 30 days, but it may be longer for you, depending on your situation. Every task you complete in this strategy gets you one step closer to improving your PR's. Go back and remember when you made that commitment to yourself. You didn't buy this book to get tucked away on your shelf and never opened again. Follow the tips. They work. You could even get some cycling buddies and do a 30-day challenge together. Then you would have an accountability partner or two.

If you are struggling here, jump on the Ride Faster Less Time Facebook page and reach out to myself or other cyclists. I want you to be successful. I want you to get faster with less time in the saddle. I want you to improve your PR's, while still spending quality time with your family and friends. If you have questions or concerns about your individual situation let's crowdsource your question and get you on track.

As you start to improve the food that you eat, your body will respond differently on the bike. You will become more fit and stronger on the bike. You will get faster. You WILL improve your PR's and achieve that goal.

Now, let's go get that goal of yours!

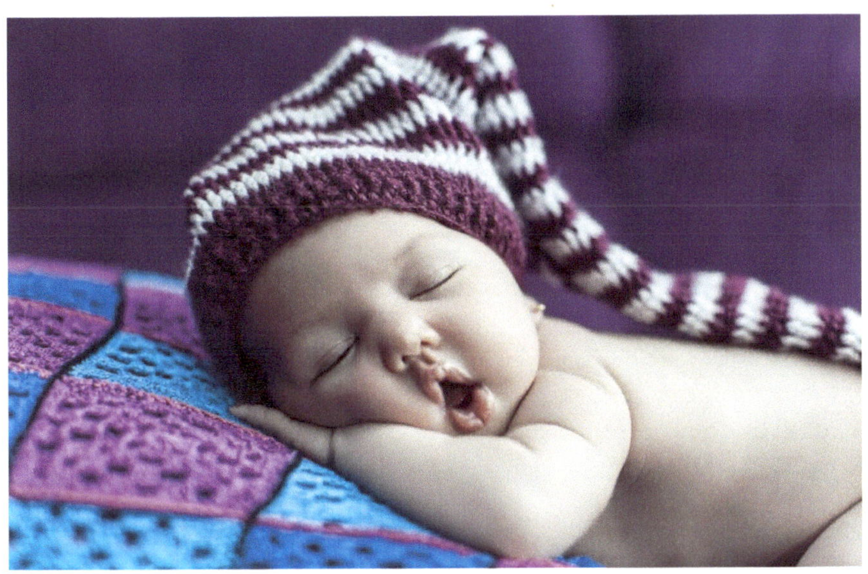

STRATEGY #2

Make Sleep a Priority

Sleep is something we all do daily. Yet, we all do it differently.
Some of us sleep like babies and others toss and turn all night. There is a
current belief that we are getting enough sleep if we can meet the following
criteria.

*We sleep the same number of hours on both work and nonwork days.
*We can awaken without an alarm clock.
*We do not use caffeine or other stimulants to remain awake or to fall
asleep.
*We do not fall asleep within 5 minutes of non-stimulating conditions.

How many of these things do you do now when you sleep?

According to the CDC, at least 1/3rd of American adults get less than the minimal recommended 7 hours of sleep per night. On average, how many hours of sleep do you get each night? We know that chronic shortened sleep cycles can lead to obesity, high blood pressure and decreased performance and alertness. If you want to improve those PR's, prioritizing your sleep is a strategy you don't want to skip.

I have heard many athletes tell me that they think lack of sleep is a "badge of honor". They think they can get much more done during the day, if they shave off some hours of sleep at night. I like to remind athletes that sleep is actually a restorative process. It helps your body repair itself from the day. It helps your brain process the day's events, somewhat like a computer clears the cache.

If we don't go into REM (Rapid Eye Movement) and deep sleep, then our brain and body do not get to fully rest and repair. We also know that chronic sleep deprivation can lead to impaired performance and alertness, as well as a host of other conditions.

Studies show that when there is a disruption of our circadian rhythms, we tend to crave more high fat and high sugar foods. Who has had sugar cravings after a night of sleep deprivation? This may be why. A study at the University of Chicago showed that when athletes slept for 6 nights with only four hours of sleep each night, they metabolized glucose less efficiently and had increased cortisol levels, which they also showed led to impaired recovery.

A study at Stanford tracked basketball players for several months. They had them add 2 more hours of sleep a night to their normal schedule. After several months, the players increased their speed by 5% and their free throws were 9% more accurate.

I have athletes that ask me all the time if sleep really makes a difference. My response is that **Sleep is for Champions**. I hope you can see that it does make a difference and choose to make sleep a priority these next 30 days.

On the next couple pages, are a list of some of the best practices to improve
your sleep. You don't have to tackle all of them in the same day. Look at the
ones that you already do and celebrate that as an accomplishment. Then
look at the practices that you are not currently following and decide the
order of those you will take on.

In the next 30 days, can you take on one of these best practices a
night, until they become a habit? It will take a commitment to get enough
sleep, just like a training schedule. It will take practice to incorporate these
sleep tips into your daily routine. But, start small with one step a night to
make them a part of your nightly routine.

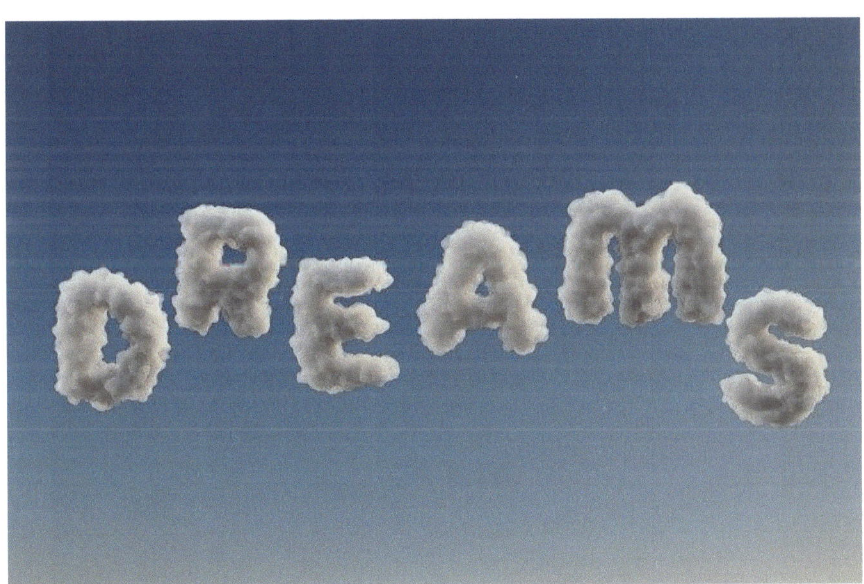

Sleep Health Best Practices

Keep a Regular Sleep Schedule

Our bodies like regularity. Try to go to bed and wake up at the same times every day. With a regular schedule, your body will know when to release calming hormones before bed and stimulating hormones to wake up.

Keep Alcohol and Caffeine to a Minimum

Both can interfere with sleep. Try to avoid caffeine within 6 hours of your bedtime. If you are sensitive to caffeine, you may need to increase the amount of time consumed before bed. Although alcohol may help you fall asleep, it usually wakes you in the middle of the night. This is due to liver enzymes metabolizing the alcohol during the night as the blood alcohol level decreases. You are then more likely to experience sleep disruptions and decreases in sleep quality.

Eat and Drink Appropriately

A regular to smallish-sized meal about 2-3 hours before bed and balanced in nutrients, can help facilitate sleep. It may be helpful to avoid spicy foods and fatty foods late at night as they may have a negative impact on your sleep.

Try not to drink too much liquid in the hours before bed, which will help you avoid waking up for bathroom breaks. If you didn't meet your hydration needs for the day, do not try and make it up right before bed. Tomorrow is a new day to get back on your hydration schedule.

Do a Brain Dump

Take a few minutes to write out a list of whatever is on your mind, before going to bed, especially those things you want to accomplish tomorrow. Whatever is on your mind, get it out and on to paper. Keep a note pad next to your bed, so if you wake up in the middle of the night and need to remember something, you can write it down and let yourself get back to sleep. You can also use a notes app or a voice recorder on your phone, if that is more your style.

Turn off Electronics or Don't Keep Them in the Bedroom

Digital devices can stimulate your brain. The recommendation is to unplug from all screens at least 60 minutes before bed. This includes television, computers and phones. The screens release a blue light that prevents our brain from preparing for sleep. If 60 minutes seems too harsh at first, try 15-20 minutes. Then move up to 30 minutes, and 45 minutes. Then you can reach 60 minutes easier. Research shows that those who have a TV in their bedroom have half as much sex as those without a TV in their bedroom. Maybe you can do your own experiment here.

Relax Before Bed

You can do this by stretching, reading or performing a meditation body scan. Develop a de-stress routine before bed that may include some yoga poses, light stretching, reading, or meditation.

Go to Bed Before Midnight

This is better aligned with natural light cycles. Plus, I can hear my father here saying, "nothing good happens after midnight". Let good sleep happen after midnight.

Sleep at Least Seven Hours Each Night

To set your bedtime, work backwards from the number of hours of sleep you want. If you need to wake up at 6 AM, 11 PM would be the latest you want to hit the pillow. This may mean you start your nighttime routine thirty minutes prior to this. Aim for your head to be on the pillow at your set bedtime.

Take a Bath or Shower or a Hot Tub Soak

A warm bath, soak or even a warm or cool shower (depending on personal preference) can promote restful sleep.

Keep Your Bedroom Dark

This means making sure your curtains and shades are not allowing light to shine through. If you can't avoid the light, you can invest in a sleep mask. If you want to use a simple hack, pull a beanie over your eyes.

Have a Stress-Free/Clutter-Free Bedroom

Get rid of stacks of mail, boxes, clothes strewn about, etc. For some, you can re-arrange your bedroom, so it is more conducive to sleep. My motto is that your bedroom should be used for sleeping and sex. Anything else is a distraction.

Keep Your Bedroom Cool

The ideal temperatures range from 60-68 F (15-20 C).

Use White Noise (if needed)

Use white noise if you have a hard time sleeping. Turn on a fan, humidifier or HEPA filter, if this will help. If the noise is distracting, then keep these devices off.

Use Aromatherapy

Some people have a better night's sleep when they use aromatherapy. Lavender is a popular essential oil that works well for sleeping. Lavender has a relaxing effect and promotes restful sleep.

If you want other ideas for utilizing aromatherapy, reach out to me on the Facebook page Ride Faster Less Time with "aromatherapy ideas or sources" in the post.

As an athlete, you are already exercising on a regular basis, which helps to improve sleep. There is a win you can count. But, one of the recommendations is to exercise at least 3 hours before bed, to not disturb your sleep health. Due to schedules, some athletes can only exercise in the evening. For most athletes, exercising in the evenings still allows them to get a good night's sleep.

For some athletes, working out too close to bedtime can keep them up. They get their endorphins going and they just can't get to sleep. If this is you and you cannot exercise at any other time but in the evening, I suggest going back to one of the sleep tips. Take a warm shower or a soak in the hot tub after exercising, but before bed. This may allow your body to relax and to have the best of both worlds.

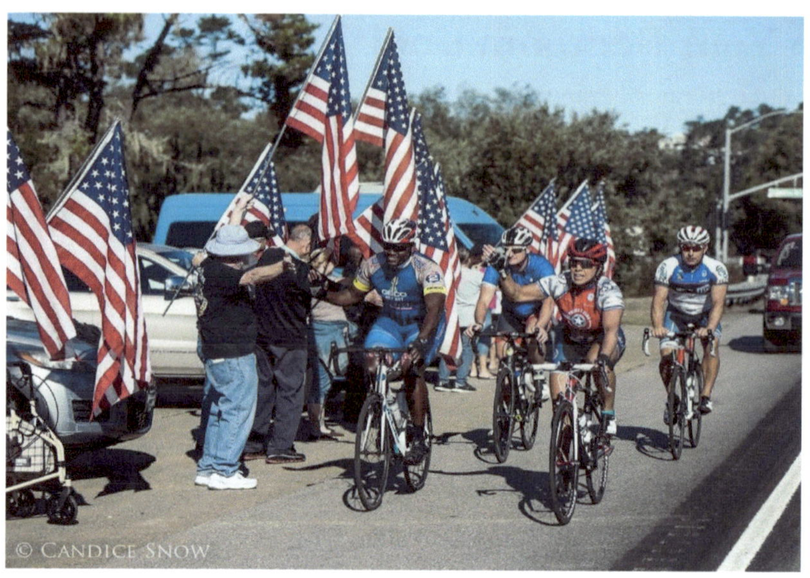

STRATEGY #3

Time Your Nutrients and Hydration ON the Bike

WHAT and WHEN you eat and drink on the bike matters. It is also important to know a couple other factors, including intensity, your speed, duration of ride and your efficiency. These other factors are all discussed in detail in our course, The Fuel Playbook and are individualized for you, the cyclist.

The important thing to keep in mind here is that every individual is different. Therefore, I am making general recommendations for you in this section. You may need to experiment and adapt these tips to your individual situation.

I am sure you have heard different recommendations on this topic. Just so you know, this topic of what to eat and when has been highly debated for years with sports nutritionists, healthcare professionals and registered dietitians.

My recommendations in here are based on many sources of science and in proven results with myself and other athletes that I have worked with over the last three decades.

You always want to experiment with food and fluids during training rides. Not on race day. When it comes to race day, you want to know that your individual eating and drinking methods are tried and true for you. It would be horrible to try a new carb drink that caused GI issues and diarrhea. No one wants diarrhea at any time, but especially not on your bike, on race day.

This strategy section may be a little more complicated, depending on your current knowledge. My intent is to explain it, so it is easy to understand, regardless of your current knowledge in this area. The term sports nutrition is the study of what you eat pre, during and post workout. As we focus on your sports nutrition during this last strategy, we want to make sure you are timing your nutrients and hydration ON the bike to get faster, gain endurance and improve those PR's.

Here is a quick, simple, generalized lesson on macronutrients and our energy systems to understand the importance of timing of nutrients. When we look at endurance sports, cycling predominantly utilizes our aerobic system. Our aerobic system relies on the breakdown of carbohydrates and fats to regenerate ATP. ATP, or Adenosine Triphosphate is the energy that drives the contraction of our muscles. Our muscles need this fuel and in aerobic exercise, our body uses the carbs and fats we have eaten and stored to create this fuel.

As cyclists, we usually over-estimate the number of calories that we need or have burned during our rides. This happens due to our electronic devices and watches estimating our caloric expenditure. I have seen this over and over again, as an athlete tells me they burned over 4000 calories on their 3-hour ride. (In reality, the best athletes in the world only burn about 1000 calories an hour for more than 3 hours and they are much more efficient than most other cyclists).

Figuring out how many calories you are burning from activity is a process. We primarily use fat and carbohydrates during aerobic exercise. We have plenty of fat stores. As a matter of fact, the average athlete can store more than 60,000 calories in fat. In the same athlete, they may only store about 2000 calories of carbohydrates or glycogen.

Glycogen is the term used for stored carbohydrates in our muscles and liver. Depending on the duration and intensity of your ride, you may burn all of your glycogen stores and therefore need to replenish with more carbohydrates along the ride. In case you are wondering, the body only uses protein as a last resort (usually extreme conditions) for fuel during aerobic exercise.

You may think it would be best to use all the fat that is stored in the body for our fuel. I wish it were that simple. But the challenge is that fat is released slow and is best utilized for low intensity exercises. As we increase our intensity and get up to 80% of our VO2Max (a measure of the maximum amount of oxygen our body can utilize during exercise), 75% of the energy used to replenish our ATP is carbohydrates. At 100% of our max, we use all carbohydrates.

As a cyclist, you will want to consume more carbohydrates to provide the fuel for your ATP needs. You may find some who disagree with this rationale and say you can tap into the fat stores. As you do become more fit, it is possible to tap into more fat stores, but my recommendation for endurance athletes is to focus more on carbohydrates to fuel those muscles. Especially when you want to improve your performance with less time in the saddle.

If you want to go into more details on how to figure out how many calories you are burning and how we can individualize your caloric deficits, then go to the end of the book and sign up for the wait list on our course, The Fuel Playbook.

Now that we finished this quick lesson, let's get to the recommendations for you ON the bike.

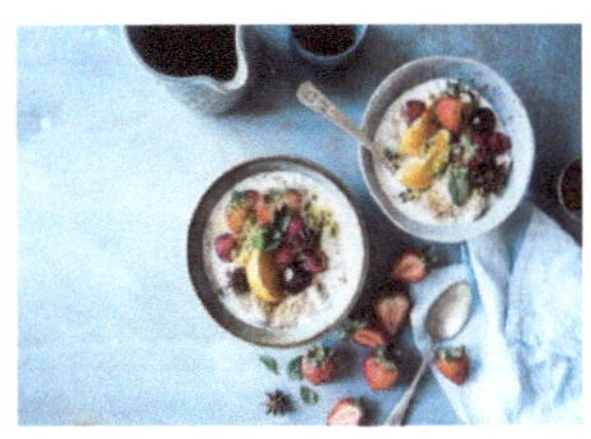

Pre-Workout

It is important to start fully fueled and hydrated on your ride. There are definitely exceptions to this, especially if you are going out for a ride that is less than 60 minutes and is low intensity. But, in general, a fueled and hydrated body is key before a workout. I would almost go so far to say that your performance on your bike depends more on your hydration levels than your food sources. But I talk about both here in an ideal situation.

The timing of your pre-ride meal or snack is important. Depending on the duration and intensity of the ride, you will want to consume a high-carbohydrate meal one to four hours prior to your ride. The overall recommendations that I practice for Endurance Athlete Nutrition is 1-4 grams of carbohydrates per kilogram (kg) of body weight in that 1-4-hour window prior to your workout.

You can also consume .3 grams of protein per kilogram of body weight with your carbohydrate meal, 1-4 hours before your workout.

A simple way to convert your body weight from pounds to kilograms is to take your weight in pounds and divide by 2.2. For example, if you weigh 150 pounds, 150 divided by 2.2= 68 kilograms. For our 150-pound (68 kg) athlete, this looks like 68-272 grams of carbohydrates in the 1-4 hours window prior to your event. (1 gram per kilogram is 68 grams and 4 grams per kilogram is 272 grams of carbohydrates). You can see a summary of different weights and recommendations in Tables 2 and 3 below.

The protein intake for this 150 lb. (68 kg) athlete would be 20 grams (rounded down from 20.4). If you have an early morning event, you may need to wake several hours before the event to make sure you are properly fueled.

This high carb meal should consist of mostly complex carbohydrates. What do complex carbohydrates look like when you eat them? They are whole grains such as brown rice, wild rice, oatmeal, whole-grain barley, bulgur (which is made from cracked wheat), and farro. One of the recommended refined grains for cyclists is white rice. It is lower in fiber, higher in carbohydrates and usually easily digested.

All of these grains can be found in your local grocery store. If you have not heard of some of them, go down the aisle with dry rice and look at your options. Other grain-like foods can include quinoa (a seed) and buckwheat (a grass). You can eat starchy vegetables including potatoes, sweet potatoes, and corn and legumes (beans, chickpeas, peas). Special note here: lentils are high in fiber. Save those until post-workout.

You will want to avoid fatty & high fiber foods prior to your workout as they may create stomach upset. Since each individual is unique, you will want to experiment to see what works best for you in this pre-ride stage. If you have a hard time eating before your ride, you can also experiment with a liquid carbohydrate drink before riding.

For hydration, we are still aiming at half of our body weight in ounces for the day. While there is not a single hydration plan that works for everyone, you can use this formula as your base. You can become dehydrated while you are sleeping, so with an early morning event, you may want to wake several hours early to also get your body hydrated. A quick glance at your urine can give you an idea if you are hydrated or not. Your urine color should look more like lemonade than apple juice for hydration. If it is darker, consume 16-24 ounces per hour to improve your hydration.

One of the most important things to consume before your ride is water. Make sure you are completely hydrated before heading out the door. The recommendation of half of your body weight is a minimum, whether you ride or not. We may need more fluid, depending on the intensity of the ride, the duration, the elements (heat, humidity), muscle mass and sweat rate (more about sweat rate later).

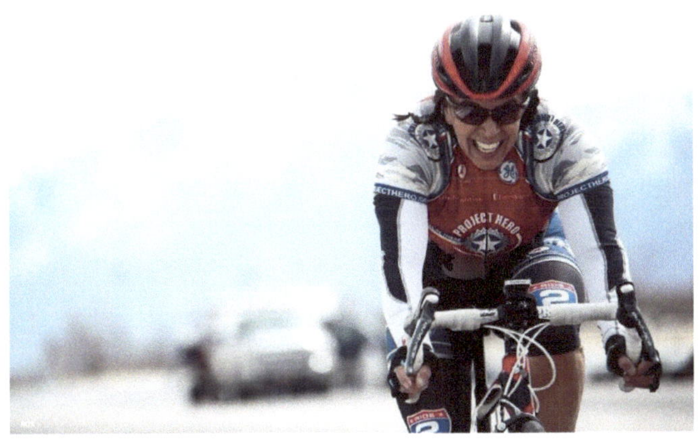

During Your Workout

If you are riding less than 60 minutes, your carbohydrate stores should be enough for your ride. For a ride less than 60 minutes, focus on your hydration. The goal is to drink one water bottle, or 16-24 ounces per hour. For less than 60 minutes, plain water should suffice. The exception to this rule would be if you are riding less than 60 minutes, but in extreme heat or humidity, or you start out dehydrated.

If you are riding for more than 60 minutes, or it is hot or humid, you will want to add in carbohydrates. I call carbohydrates the "master fuel". The "gas for an athlete's tank". As carbohydrates are oxidized at rates up to 1 gram per hour, you will want to aim for approximately 30-60 grams of carbohydrates per hour, for events lasting between one hour and less than 2.5 hours in duration.

The recommendation for Endurance Athletes for rides lasting more than 2.5 hours is 60-70 grams per hour. (Elite cyclists have trained their systems to process up to 90 grams of carbohydrates per hour, by combining different combinations of carbohydrates, so if you have heard this larger number, that is possible.) It is not something we will cover in this book.

There are some quick sources of carbohydrates in gels or chews, if you can tolerate them. You can also put a carbohydrate/hydration drink in one of your water bottles, if it is easier to drink your carbs while on the bike.

If you want to know my favorite hydration carb drink put a post in the Ride Faster Less Time Facebook Group and I will give you my carb drink recommendation. You can also use real food and put a banana in your pocket (approx. 27 grams of carbs) or some dates (18 grams of carbs per date) or dried fruit (25 grams in 1 ounce) in a plastic bag to carry with you. I love to eat real food on the bike, as my body seems to respond better on the bike. My favorite on the bike combo is dried mangos and dates. As a reminder, this is a process to experiment with during your training rides.

Pre-assess the duration of your ride and pre-fill 2 bottles if you will be riding more than 60 minutes. Fill one bottle with plain water and one bottle with a carbohydrate/hydration drink mix. If you will be out riding for more than 2 hours, plan to stop at a water stop to refill your bottles. You may also want to carry a carbohydrate hydration packet with you if you will be on the road for more than 2 hours.

If your riding event is high intensity, we can add some protein into the mix. The recommendation for high intensity events is to take in .25 grams of protein per kilogram of body weight per hour of the event. If we had a 4-hour bike race, with our 150 lb. (68 kg) athlete described above, this would equate to 17 grams of protein per hour for this high intensity event. Most athletes will supplement with a liquid protein supplement to get this in, but other options may be a nut butter sandwich with honey or banana, or a famous rice cake with peanut butter and jelly. Look at Table 4 & Table 5 to see examples of real food and grams of protein and carbohydrates per food item.

Studies have shown that adding protein to a carbohydrate beverage during exhaustive endurance exercise suppresses markers of muscle damage post exercise and decreases muscular soreness. They also show that adding protein to carbohydrate consumption throughout a prolonged bout of endurance exercise promotes a higher whole-body net protein balance.

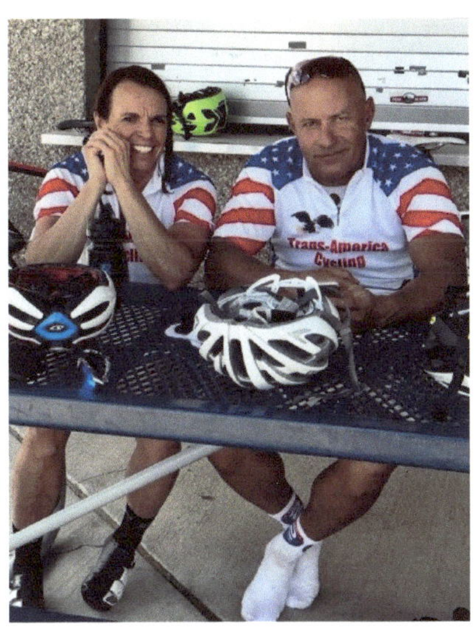

Post Workout

It is important to start rebuilding your depleted glycogen stores immediately after exercise. Your goal is to consume 1.2 grams of carbohydrates per kilogram of body weight in the two hours post workout. Taking our example above for our 150-pound (68 kg) athlete, the carbohydrate goal for this cyclist is 81.6 or rounded up to 82 grams of carbohydrates over the next two hours post workout. (68 x 1.2−81.6).

You will also want to consume .3 gram of protein for every kilogram of body weight within two hours post workout. To calculate this, use the example that we used above in pre-workout protein consumption. (.3x68=20.4) You can round down to 20 grams of protein in the two hours post workout. This would be equivalent to approximately a palm-sized lean meat serving.

The ideal scenario is to time your ride before your meal (breakfast, lunch or dinner). Then you can get off your bike and eat a healthy meal to replenish your body with these recommended consumptions. If that is not possible, eat as soon as possible post ride, but within 2 hours of ending your ride.

Adding a little sodium (300-500 mg) to your meal or in a post hydration drink will help with rehydration. You can also calculate your sweat rate by weighing yourself naked before and after your workout. Aim to rehydrate with 16-24 ounces of fluid for every pound lost during your workout.

Think of food as a team effort. In team sports, you know that you are only as good as your team is, right? When you do not provide all of the right nutrients to your body or limit them, they cannot perform as a team and then the overall whole suffers.

You are on a mission to improve your overall endurance, improve your performance and improve those personal records on the bike. The timing and intake of your nutrients and hydration ON the bike is a key part of this mission. It takes a few calculations, but once you get them in place, you are ready to roll.

Check out Tables 2 & 3 to find your individual numbers. If all these calculations have you second guessing yourself, then head on over to the sign up for our course, The Fuel Playbook. We will personalize these calculations and design a plan just for you.

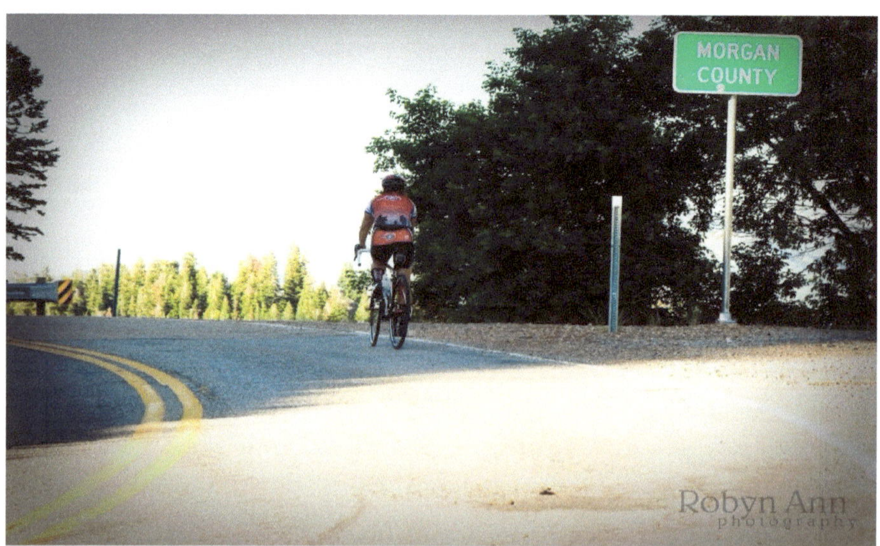

Table 1. Summary of Nutrient and Hydration Timing

This table summarizes the nutrients and hydration timing and amount pre, during and post event.

	Pre	During	Post
Carbs	1-4g/kg (1-4 hrs. pre event)	30-60 g/hour <2.5 hours 60-70 g/hour >2.5 hours	1.2 g/kg within 2 hours post event,
Protcin	.3g/kg with carbs	.25g/kg/h in high intensity cvcnts	.3g/kg with carbs
Water	1 water bottle 1 hour prior to event. (16-24 ounces).	1 water bottle per hour min. (16-24 ounces)	16-20 ounces per lb. lost. Weigh self before and after during training.

American College of Sports Medicine (ACSM) and International Society of Sports Nutrition (ISSN) combined recommendations.

Table 2. Carbohydrate Intake: Pre, During and Post

Weight (WT) in lbs.	WT converted to KG (rounded) Wt./2.2	Carbs Pre- 1-4g/kg 1-4 hrs. pre	Carbs During 30-60 g/hr.<2.5 hrs. 60-70g/hr.>2.5 hrs.	Carbs Post 1.2g/kg in 2 hrs. (rounded)
110	50	50-200 g	30-60g or 60-70g/hr.	60 g
130	59	59-236 g	30-60g or 60-70g/hr.	71 g
150	68	68-272 g	30-60g or 60-70g/hr.	82 g
170	77	77-308 g	30-60g or 60-70g/hr.	92 g
190	86	86-344 g	30-60g or 60-70g/hr.	103 g
210	95	95-380 g	30-60g or 60-70g/hr.	114 g
220	100	100-400 g	30-60g or 60-70g/hr.	120 g
240	109	109-436 g	30-60g or 60-70g/hr.	131 g
260	118	118-472 g	30-60g or 60-70g/hr.	142 g
280	127	127-508 g	30-60g or 60-70g/hr.	152 g

The Fuel Trainer 2020

Table 3. Protein Intake: Pre, During and Post

Weight (WT) in lbs.	WT converted to KG (rounded) Wt./2.2	Protein Pre- .3g/kg w carbs (rounded)	Protein During Only w high intensity .25g/kg/hr.	Protein Post .3g/kg w carbs (rounded)
110	50	15 g	12 g	15 g
130	59	18 g	15 g	18 g
150	68	20 g	17 g	20 g
170	77	23 g	19 g	23 g
190	86	26 g	21 g	26 g
210	95	28 g	24 g	28 g
220	100	30 g	25 g	30 g
240	109	33 g	27 g	33 g
260	118	35 g	29 g	35 g
280	127	38 g	32 g	38 g

Created by: The Fuel Trainer 2020

Table 4. Common Foods and Carbohydrate Content

Food Name	Amount of Food	Grams of Carbs
Apple	1 med.	25
Banana	1 med.	27
Beets	1 cup	13
Dates	1	18
Fig	1	8
Garbanzo Beans	1 cup	21
Kidney Beans	1 cup	19
Mango	1 cup fresh	25
Milk	1 cup	12
Pasta	½ cup	20
Potato	1 med	37
Quinoa	1 cup	40
Sweet Potato	1 med.	24
Rice	1 cup	45
Yogurt	1 small container	6

The Fuel Trainer 2020

Table 5. Common Foods and Protein Content

Food Name	Amount of Food	Grams of Protein
Black Beans	½ cup	8
Cheese	1 stick	6
Chicken Breast	3 oz.	24
Cottage Cheese	½ cup	12
Edamame	½ cup	9
Egg	1 whole	6
Greek Yogurt	7 oz. container	20
Hemp Seeds	3 TBL	10
Kefir	1 cup	10
Lentils	½ cup	9
Milk (Cow)	1 cup	8
Peanut Butter	2 TBL	8
Pumpkin Seeds	¼ cup	10
Salmon	3 oz.	19
Tempeh	3 oz.	16
Turkey Breast	1 oz slice	8
Tuna	6.5 oz can	31

The Fuel Trainer 2020

After the 30 Days

Congratulations!

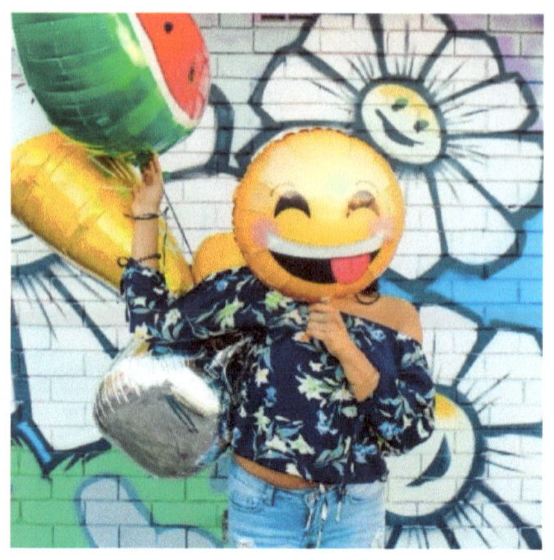

You have followed this plan for the last 30 days and it is time to celebrate. Let's start by looking at your times on the bike. Pull out your spreadsheet that we created in the beginning and let's look at those numbers. Let's take a look at your Achievements. How did you do? Which segments improved? What was your biggest improvement? Do you feel that you have developed a habit with these strategies?

Let's stop and acknowledge your accomplishments these last 30 days. You stuck to your plan and improved your personal records (PR's). Great job! You set out to accomplish a goal and you did it.

Make sure you share your success with your family and support team. They have been there to support you the entire time and they will also want to share in your success. Share your success with other riders. Let them know how you improved your PR's, while still maintaining quality family time and a healthy life off the bike. They probably have already noticed and may have said something to you already. They may have asked you what you are doing. Share your success story with them so they can celebrate your accomplishments with you. You can even share how they can get this book, (as long as they are a teammate and not your opponent, ha-ha), so they can also learn to get faster without less time in the saddle.

What is next? Where do you go from here? The good news is that you can take these same strategies and apply them for the next 3 months. You have consistently followed these strategies for the last 30 days and have created successful habits. It will be easier to continue applying them until you are ready to go to the next level. You will also find that your support team has adapted to these strategies and it will be easier for them to continue working on them with you.

If you were not as diligent these last 30 days, go back and repeat the 30 days. Go back and follow each strategy. The strategies will work, if you follow them. If you are having challenges or are choosing "overwhelm", then message me on the Facebook page. Let's talk about your challenges.

As you look forward to the next three months, if you are ready for an additional challenge, you can take your strategies to the next level, with the steps listed on the next page.

If you want more accountability and a supportive group, you may be ready for our 6-week course, The Fuel Playbook: Strategies for Endurance Athletes to discover the keys to unlocking the power of nutrition to fuel their bodies for optimal athletic performance. If you are ready for a personalized plan in a supportive environment with other Endurance Athletes, then sign up now for our course Wait List.

Why should you take this course?

- Take the Guess Work out of What to Eat Before, During and After a Workout for YOUR Individual Needs
- Boost your Endurance
- Become More Efficient in your Sport
- Live a Balanced and Healthy Life as an Athlete
- Focus on your Specific Needs for your personalized goals
- Set your own SMART Goals
- Get the Ins and Outs of Supplements and know IF you Really Need Them
- Improve your Athletic Performance
- Improve Recovery Time
- Increase your Confidence in your Sport
- Eat simple foods from the Grocery Store and your Kitchen
- Learn Tasty New Recipes to Cook
- Improve your Everyday Health
- Have more Energy during the Season and the off-season
- Led by Dr. Lorri Zenoni and based on nutritional and lifestyle science. NO guessing if it is reliable information.

Specific steps to move forward, post 30 Days

- Increase your fruits and vegetable intake to 3-4 servings of fruit and 4-6 servings of vegetables a day. Your fist is equivalent to a serving.
- Aim for eating 1.4-1.6 grams of protein per kilogram of body weight every day. For our 150 lb. (68 kg) athlete, this is 95-109 grams per day. You can break that up per meal with a goal of approximately 24-27 grams per meal. This is a general recommendation from the ISSN (International Society of Sports Nutrition). As we discussed, your individual needs may be different. You can set up an individualized consult or you can join our course, The Fuel Playbook, for a more personalized plan.
- Continue with a new vegetable recipe each week. Enlist your family to pick out a vegetable. Consider making it a family game that an assigned family member makes a new vegetable recipe once a week.
- Reduce fast food visits to no more than twice a month. If you do visit, make it an intentional visit and know what you are having before you go.
- Eliminate soda and sweetened drinks and save for special occasions only.
- Maintain water intake to half of your body weight in ounces and up to your entire body weight in ounces depending on conditions (heat, humidity, riding your bike for longer rides).
- Continue to eat regularly throughout the day, aiming for at least 3-4 meals and 1-2 snacks a day.
- Continue to focus on eating slowly and being more mindful of the number of chews per bite as well as what you are putting in your body. Eat with a partner and put your utensils down and have an extended conversation with them over your meal.

- Continue to make sleep a priority. Tell yourself that "Sleep is for Champions". Continue until all the best practices are a part of your nightly routine.
- Continue to dial in the timing and substance of your nutrients and hydration on your bike. Do you know what works best for you? Keep experimenting until you find the right combination for you.

> **Bonus tip: Remember to Drink Your Water**
>
> Here is a way to remember to drink your water daily.
> *Find a container that is easy to carry around.
> *Measure how many ounces it holds. Determine your ideal water intake each day by dividing your weight by 2. For example, if you weigh 150 pounds, you will aim for 75 ounces of water each day.
> If your water container holds 25 ounces, you will need to fill it 3 times each day to meet your 75 ounces daily recommendation. You will need one less rubber band than how many times you will need to fill.
> Fill your container first thing in the morning and put 2 rubber bands on the water container. You can put them on the neck of the container or around the bottom. Once you have drunk the water in the container, re-fill it and take off a rubber band. Continue until there are no more rubber bands left on the container.
> *You can put the used rubber bands on your wrist to re-use for tomorrow or on a different part of the bottle than started.

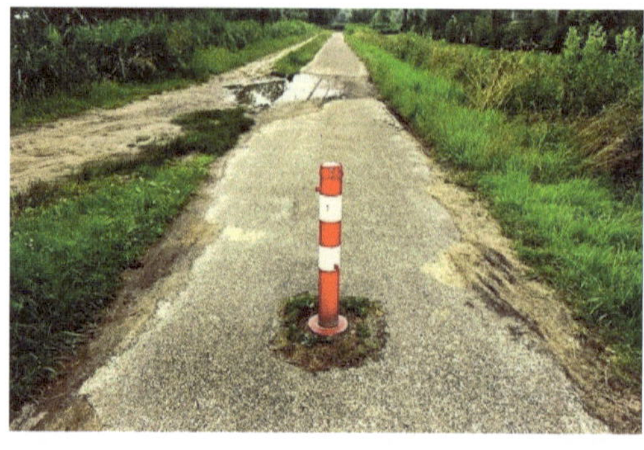

Breaking Down the Roadblocks

After the 30 days, you may want to go back to your old habits. You may have looked at this as a 30-day challenge only and not a lifestyle change. But, ask yourself these questions. Are you going to keep riding your bike? I'm almost certain the answer is yes. Do you want to continue to improve your personal records on your bike? I'm pretty sure that is another yes. So, look at these strategies in this book as changes for a lifetime. Not just a quick, 30-Day challenge. You may not make as large gains as you did these last 30 days, but you WILL continue to improve on your bike, with less training time, IF you stick with these strategies.

It may have been easier for you to focus on 30 days. Most people say they can do anything for 30 days. As you look at taking this plan outside of 30 days, you may have questions for particular situations. I have taken a few of the most asked questions and given a few tips for those situations.

Will these strategies help me lose weight?

While you may lose weight with these strategies, this is not a weight loss program. The strategies in this book are designed to help you improve your health and therefore, improve your performance on the bike. I recommend that if you want to lose weight, you focus on that during your off season. The time to dial in your nutrition and improve your body composition (more lean muscle and less fat) is during the off season. For most cyclists, the off season is in the winter months. But it may be different for you. If weight loss is a specific goal for you, then join me for a more personalized plan in The Fuel Playbook course.

What about when I go out to eat?

Going out to eat is going to happen. Just as life celebrations are going to happen. (birthdays, anniversaries, etc.) But you can plan for it. Plan ahead of time WHAT you are going to eat at the restaurant. Are you splitting a meal, sharing a meal, ordering something that will heat up well tomorrow or ordering a smaller portion? Plan before you get there, so you know exactly what you are having when you do go out to eat.

If you have not been there before, go online and look up their menu. Find a healthy meal that you can eat. Look at reviews. Do they have big portions? If so, plan to take half home or share a meal. Order water as your main drink. Aim to drink a whole glass of water before you start eating anything. This will help to hydrate your body and create an environment where you are less likely to overeat.

Remember you are there for the company and to foster your relationships. Enjoy the people around you. Enjoy the conversations and the interactions. Yes, we also go out to eat because we enjoy the food. So, enjoy the food. Enjoy every bite. Slow down and savor each bite. Put your utensils down in between bites, so you can intentionally slow down your eating. All of these tips can help you enjoy your time out to eat, yet not get too derailed from your plan.

What about in the winter when I am riding indoors, instead of outside?

Depending on your geographical location, you may be able to ride outside all year long, while others are stuck inside on an indoor trainer during the winter. Others prefer an indoor trainer at any time of the year. No matter how and where you ride, either on an indoor trainer or on the road, you can still apply these strategies. If you spend all winter indoors, or you ride mostly on an indoor trainer, you may want to get your vitamin D levels checked. If you want to get them checked and do not want to pay an expensive copay, then check out Dr. Lorri's lab site. We have affordable lab testing available to our readers. Check out our lab site here: https://www.ultalabtests.com/fueltrainer

I am going on vacation and my sleep patterns will change for that week. What is the best advice for prioritizing my sleep when on vacation?

I love traveling and my husband and I do it often. So, I know that when you are in a new city, there is so much you want to do and see, that your sleep may be impacted. My advice? Enjoy your travels and vacation. You may not be able to stay up until the wee hours of the night every night and expect to be bright eyed and bushy tailed in the morning, but you also may never be in this city again. Listen to your heart and your body. See the sights you want. Go to the 10 PM show, have dessert at midnight and live your best life while on vacation. Keep to the principles as much as possible while away and then get right back to them when you return home.

Why is whey protein recommended over others?

Supplementing with whey protein provides a distinct advantage over other protein sources on muscle protein synthesis. Whey protein contains an array of biologically active peptides whose amino acid sequences give them specific signaling effects to support muscle maintenance, muscle adaption, and quality of sleep for improved recovery.

If you cannot tolerate dairy, or want a plant-based option, then let's explore other options. There are plenty of plant-based protein powders made with pea or brown rice or mung beans. You can also choose non-dairy milks to mix with the plant protein for added protein such as almond, cashew, rice, coconut, oat or macadamia nut. The beauty is that you can find all of these non-dairy milk options in most grocery stores now.

Does caffeine improve my performance and if so, how much do I need?

There are inconsistencies in studies that look at enhanced athletic performance after ingestion of caffeine. This is another area to experiment with your own findings.

One result of a study suggests that high intensity cycling performance can be increased following moderate caffeine ingestion and that it may be related to a reduction in RPE (Rate of Perceived Exertion) and an elevation in blood lactate concentration. The amount of caffeine that was used in this particular study was 5 mg/kg of body weight. In our 150 lb. athlete (68 kg) example, this would equate to 340 mg.

For reference, an average cup of regular black coffee has approximately 95 mg per cup, depending on how it is brewed. This is about 3.5 cups of coffee. Other study recommendations give an upper limit of 3 mg/kg of body weight. This would equate to approximately 204 mgs of caffeine, or approximately 2.5 cups of coffee. My recommendation is to experiment during training with the lowest amount that will provide the results you are seeking.

What if my PR's do not improve?

I would go back and look at your strategies. Have you been following them? Have you taken the strategies seriously or just half-hearted? If you have been following them diligently and are not improving, then reach out to me at the Ride Faster Less Time Facebook page. This page is here for you. We will dissect your actions and see what is happening in your particular case.

People who train with me often ask, "how do I sustain these changes"? I say to go back to the basics and look at them as changes for a lifetime, not just a quick fix. If you need to go back and follow the 30-Day plan, then do that. If you have other questions that come up, join me on the Facebook page, *Ride Faster Less Time* and ask your questions there.

If you want to continue to ride your bike and maintain your PR's, you will find a way to keep up the healthy eating, prioritize your sleep and continue to time your nutrients and hydration on your bike.

If you want to take it to the next level, with personalized coaching, then join our Wait List for our 6-week course, The Fuel Playbook. We will provide strategies for the Endurance Athlete to unlock the power of nutrition and fuel their bodies for optimal athletic performance.

Keep the Rubber Side Down

Thank you for allowing me to be on this journey with you. I know that these strategies have worked for me and countless others that I have coached. I was excited to put this in a book format that others could benefit from. The intent was to make it simple and easy to follow.

We are all at different places in our journey and all of our bodies respond differently to training regiments. Yet, I wanted you, the cyclist, to be able to pick up this book and have it as a simple read, a simple plan, yet make a difference in your life. I want your cycling life to be fun and exciting while still living the life you want off the bike. I have found it is possible and hope you find that as well.

I'd love to hear about your success stories. I love to know that others can ride their bike and enjoy the many other aspects of their life off the bike. When I reach out to you, please know that I want to hear your story. I want to know how this book has helped you. If you have any comments or suggestions, I would also love to hear from you. Please feel free to reach out to me on our Ride Faster Less Time Facebook page. I look forward to connecting with you.

Now go get those PR's!

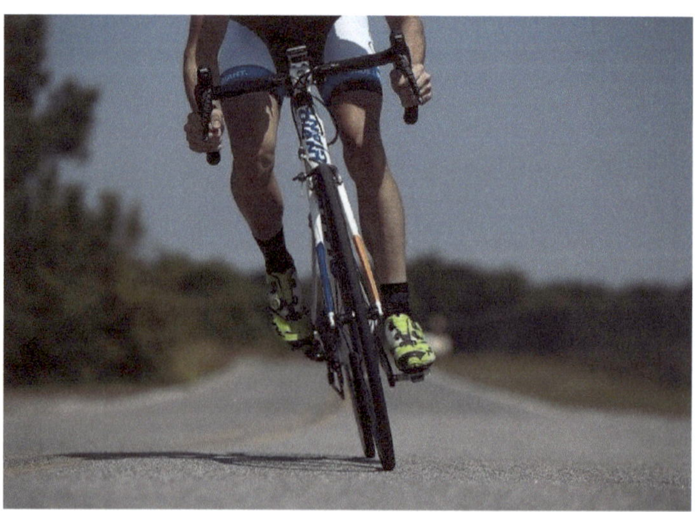

<u>Ready for More?</u>

Now that you know the basics of how to ride
    faster with less time in the saddle, are you
ready for a more personalized program?

Are you Ready to take it to the Next Level?

   We offer a 6-Week Course titled: The Fuel
Playbook: Strategies for Endurance Athletes to
discover the keys to unlocking the power
of nutrition and fuel their bodies for Optimal
                Athletic Performance.

We only release this course two times a year.
    If you want to get on the Wait List for this
                Course, please email me at
           drlorriz@thefueltrainer.com

Put *The Fuel Playbook* in the subject line to take
your performance to the next level.

References

- Kushida, CA. Sleep Deprivation: Basic Science, Physiology, Behavior. 2005. Marcel Dekker.
- Ansch, Browman, Mitler and Walsh. Sleep: A Scientific Perspective (1988)
- Jäger R, Kerksick CM, Campbell BI et al. International Society of Sports Nutrition Position Stand: protein and exercise. J Int Soc Sports Nutr. 2017 Jun 20; 14:20.
- Antonio J, Ellerbroek A, Silver T et al. A high protein diet (3.4 g/kg/d) combined with a heavy resistance training program improves body composition in healthy trained men and women—a follow-up investigation. J Int Soc Sports Nutr. 2015 Oct 20; 12:39.
- Antonio J, Ellerbroek A, Silver T et al. The effects of a high protein diet on indices of health and body composition—a crossover trial in resistance-trained men. J Int Soc Sports Nutr. 2016 Jan 16; 13:3.
- Antonio J, Ellerbroek A, Silver T et al. A high protein diet has no harmful effects: a one-year crossover study in resistance-trained males. J Nutr Metab. 2016; 2016:9104792.
- Antonio J, Peacock CA, Ellerbroek A et al. The effects of consuming a high protein diet (4.4 g/kg/d) on body composition in resistance-trained individuals. J Int Soc Sports Nutr. 2014 May 12; 11:19.
- Wolfe RR, Cifelli AM, Kostas G et al. Optimizing protein intake in adults: interpretation and application of the recommended dietary allowance compared with the acceptable macronutrient distribution range. Adv Nutr. 2017 Mar 15;8(2):266-275
- Andersen LL, Tufekovic G, Zebis MK et al. The effect of resistance training combined with timed ingestion of protein on muscle fiber size and muscle strength. Metab Clin Exp. 2005 Feb;54(2):151-6.
- Burke DG, Chilibeck PD, Davidson KS et al. The effect of whey protein supplementation with and without creatine monohydrate combined with resistance training on lean tissue mass and muscle strength. Int J Sport Nutr Exerc Metab. 2001 Sep;11(3):349-64.
- Hulmi JJ, Kovanen V, Selanne H et al. Acute and long-term effects of resistance exercise with or without protein ingestion on muscle hypertrophy and gene expression. Amino Acids. Jul;37(2):297308.

- Kerksick CM, Rasmussen CJ, Lancaster SL et al. The effects of protein and amino acid supplementation on performance and training adaptations during ten weeks of resistance training. J Strength Cond Res. 2006 Aug;20(3):643-53
- Candow DG, Burke NC, Smith-Palmer T et al. Effect of whey and soy protein supplementation combined with resistance training in young adults. Int J Sport Nutr Exerc Metab. 2006 Jun;16(3):23344.
- Cribb PJ, Williams AD, Stathis CG et al. Effects of whey isolate, creatine, and resistance training on muscle hypertrophy. Med Sci Sports Exerc. 2007 Feb;39(2):298-307.
- Areta JL, Burke LM, Ross ML et al. Timing and distribution of protein ingestion during prolonged recovery from resistance exercise alters myofibrillar protein synthesis. J Physiol. 2013 May 1;591(9):2319-31
- Arciero PJ, Ives SJ, Norton C et al. Protein-Pacing and MultiComponent Exercise Training Improves Physical Performance Outcomes in Exercise-Trained Women: The PRISE 3 Study. Nutrients. 2016 Jun 1;8(6).
- Ives SJ, Norton C, Miller V et al. Multi-modal exercise training and protein-pacing enhances physical performance adaptations independent of growth hormone and BDNF but may be dependent on IGF-1 in exercise-trained men. Growth Horm IGF Res. 2017 Feb; 32:60-70.
- Tang JE, Moore DR, Kujbida GW et al. Ingestion of whey hydrolysate, casein, or soy protein isolate: effects on mixed muscle protein synthesis at rest and following resistance exercise in young men. J App Physiol. 2009 Sep;107(3):987-92.
- West DW, Burd NA, Coffey VG et al. Rapid aminoacidemia enhances myofibrillar protein synthesis and anabolic intramuscular signaling responses after resistance exercise. Am J Clin Nutr. 2011 Sep;94(3):795-803.
- Staples AW, Burd NA, West DW et al. Carbohydrate does not augment exercise-induced protein accretion versus protein alone. Med Sci Sports Exerc. Med Sci Sports Exerc. 2011 Jul;43(7):115461.
- Markus CR, Olivier B, De Haan EH. Whey protein rich in alphalactalbumin increases the ratio of plasma tryptophan to the sum of the other large neutral amino acids and improves cognitive performance in stress-vulnerable subjects. Am J Clin Nutr. 2002 Jun;75(6):1051-6.
- Minet-Ringuet J, Le Ruyet PM, Tome D et al. A tryptophan-rich protein diet efficiently restores sleep after food deprivation in the rat. Behav Brain Res. 2004 Jul 9;152(2):335-40.

- Jonathon D. Wiles, Damian Coleman, Michael Tegerdine & Ian L. Swaine (2006) The effects of caffeine ingestion on performance time, speed and power during a laboratory based 1km cycling time-trial, Journal of Sport Sciences, 24:11, 1165-1171.
- Higgins, S; Straight, C.R; Lewis, R.D. The effects of Pre-Exercise Caffeinated-coffee Ingestion on Endurance Performance, An Evidence-Based Review. Int. J. Sports Nutr Exerc. Metab. 2016, 26, 221-239.
- Southward K, Rutherfurd-Markwick KJ, Ali A. The Effect of Acute Caffeine Ingestion on Endurance Performance: A Systematic Review and Meta-Analysis. Sports Med. 2018 Aug; 48 (8): 19131928.
- Washington State University: "How Sleep Affects Sports Performance". Taheri, S. PLoS Medicine, December 2004.
- American Academy of Sleep Medicine. "Extra Sleep Improves Athletic Performance." ScienceDaily. ScienceDaily, 10 June 2008.
- Waterhouse, J. Atkinson, G. Edwards, B, Reilly, T. J. "Naps and Athletic Performance". Sports Sci. 2007, Dec 25(14): 1557-66.
- "Testosterone levels in reduced sleep". JAMA, 2011;305(21) 2173-2174
- "Circadian Rhythm Disruption Study". Rush University Medical Center, 2014.

NOTES

www.ingramcontent.com/pod-product-compliance
Lightning Source LLC
Chambersburg PA
CBHW040227240726
48664CB00001B/33